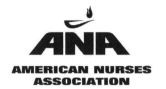

AMERICAN NURSES
ASSOCIATION

D0477759

# Safe Patient Handling and Mobility: Interprofessional National Standards

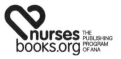

nurses
books.org THE PUBLISHING PROGRAM OF ANA

American Nurses Association
Silver Spring, Maryland
2013

The American Nurses Association (ANA) is a national professional association. This ANA publication—*Safe Patient Handling and Mobility: Interprofessional National Standards*—reflects the thinking of the practice specialty of holistic nursing on various issues and should be reviewed in conjunction with state board of nursing policies and practices. State law, rules, and regulations govern the practice of nursing, while *Safe Patient Handling and Mobility: Interprofessional National Standards* guides nurses in the application of their professional skills and responsibilities.

**American Nurses Association**
8515 Georgia Avenue, Suite 400
Silver Spring, MD 20910-3492
1-800-274-4ANA
www.NursingWorld.org

**Published by Nursesbooks.org**
The Publishing Program of ANA
www.Nursesbooks.org/

ISBN: 978-1-55810-519-5     SAN: 851-3481     08/2013R

First printing June 2013. Second printing August 2013.

# Contents

# Contributors

## Work Group

### Mary W. Matz, MSPH, CPE, CSPHP – Chair
National Program Manager, Patient Care Ergonomics
Occupational Health Strategic Healthcare Group, Office of Public Health
Veterans Health Administration

### *Work Group Members*

### Mary Bliss, RN, COHN
Association of Occupational Health Professionals in Healthcare
Board Member
Coordinator of Employee Health Services
Methodist Medical Center

### Myrna C. Callison, COL, SPPhD, OTR/L, AEP
OT Consultant to the Army Surgeon General
Asst. Chief, Army Medical Specialist Corps
Occupational Health Sciences Portfolio Executive Officer
U. S. Army Public Health Command

### Mary Carr, RN, MPH
Associate Director for Regulatory Affairs
National Association for Home Care & Hospice

### Colleen Christopher, BS, OTR
*Sub-Group Chair*
Clinical Consultant
Diligent Guaranteed Solutions
ArjoHuntleigh, Getinge Group

## James W. Collins, PhD, MSME
Associate Director for Science, Division of Safety Research
Centers for Disease Control and Prevention
The National Institute for Occupational Safety and Health

## Amy Darragh, PhD, OTR/L
*Sub-Group Chair*
American Occupational Therapy Association  Representative
School of Health and Rehabilitation Sciences
The Wexner Medical Center
The Ohio State University

## Lena L. Deter, RN, MPH, CSPHP
Clinical Consultant
DELHEC, LLC

## Lynda Enos, RN, MS, COHN-S, CPE
*Sub-Group Chair*
American Association of Safe Patient Handling and Movement Representative
Certified Professional Ergonomist
Ergonomics/Human Factors Consultant
HumanFit, LLC

## Guy Fragala, PhD, PE, CSP, CSPHP
Senior Advisor for Ergonomics
Patient Safety Center of Inquiry
Veterans Health Administration

## Genevieve Gipson, RN, MEd, RNC
Director, National Network of Nursing Assistants

## Kenneth J. Harwood, PT, PhD, CIE
*Sub-Group Chair*
Associate Professor
Clinical Research and Leadership
Program in Physical Therapy
George Washington University

## Bill Hirschuber, MA, OTR/L
Ergonomics and Safe Patient Handling Coordinator, Case Manager
Employee Occupational Health & Safety
Park Nicollet Health Services

**Ninica (Niki) Howard, MSc, CPE**
Senior Researcher
SHARP Program
Washington Department of Labor and Industries

**Dee Kumpar, RN, BSN, MBA, CSPHP**
Director, Safe Lifting Programs and Services
Hill-Rom

**Kelsey L. McCoskey, MS, OTR/L, CPE, CSPHP**
*Sub-Group Chair*
Ergonomist
U.S. Army Public Health Command
Army Institute of Public Health

**Marsha Medlin, MPA, RN**
President, Safe Lifting Solutions

**Vivian B. Miller, BA, CPHQ, LHRM, CPHRM, DFASHRM**
Quality, Risk and Compliance Consultant
Washington Hospital Center OutPatient Behavioral Health Services

**Mary J. Ogg, MSN, RN, CNOR**
Perioperative Nursing Specialist
Association of periOperative Registered Nurses – Representative

**Gail Powell-Cope, PhD, RN, FAAN**
Associate Director, VA Patient Safety Center of Inquiry
James A. Haley Veterans Hospital

**Rich Schleckser, ARM, NEBOSH, CMIOSH, CSPHP**
*Sub-Group Chair*
Senior Risk Control Service Director
Liberty Mutual Insurance Company

**Lori Severson, MS, HEM, ASP**
Senior Loss Control Consultant
Lockton Companies

**Deborah L. Spratt, MPA, BSN, RN, CNOR, NEA-BC CRCST, CHL**
President, Association of periOperative Registered Nurses

**Bob Williamson, RN, BSN, MS, CWCP**
Director, Associate Safety
Ascension Health

**Donna Zankowski, RN, COHN**
*Sub-Group Chair*
American Association of Occupational Health Nurses – Representative
Occupational Nurse Case Manager
Corporate Occupational Health Solutions

## ANA Staff

**Suzy Harrington, DNP, RN, MCHES**
Director
Department for Health, Safety, and Wellness

**Jaime Murphy Dawson, MPH**
Senior Policy Analyst
Department for Health, Safety, and Wellness

**Maureen E. Cones, Esq.**
Associate General Counsel
Credentialing, Litigation, Nursing Practice
Office of General Counsel

**Carol J. Bickford, PhD, RN-BC, CPHIMS**
Senior Policy Fellow
Department of Nursing Practice and Policy

## Acknowledgments

**Colin J. Brigham, CIH, CSP, CPE, CPEA, CSPHP**
President of Association of Safe Patient Handling Professionals
Vice President of 1 Source Safety & Health Inc.

**Susan Gallagher, PhD, MSN, RN, WOCN, CBN, HCRM, CSPHP**
Celebration Institute, Inc.

**Ed Hall, MS, CSP**
Chief Operating Officer
Stanford University Medical Network Risk Authority

## Ron Romano, RN

American Association of Safe Patient Handling and Movement – Representative
Founder and Vice President of Professional Services
American Association for Long Term Care Nursing

### *Technical Writer*

## Amy Garcia, MSN, RN, CAE

Independent consultant

*ANA wishes to thank the contributors for generously giving their time and expertise to the development of this document. We would like to specially acknowledge our chairperson, Mary Matz, for her leadership and dedication to safe patient handling and mobility.*

## About the American Nurses Association

The American Nurses Association (ANA) is the only full-service professional organization representing the interests of the nation's 3.1 million registered nurses through its constituent/state nurses association and its organizational affiliates. The ANA advances the nursing profession by fostering high standards of nursing practice, promoting the rights of nurses in the workplace, projecting a positive and realistic view of nursing, and by lobbying the Congress and regulatory agencies on healthcare issues affecting nurses and the public.

## About Nursesbooks.org

Nursesbooks.org publishes books on ANA core issues and programs, including ethics, leadership, quality, specialty practice, advanced practice, and the profession's enduring legacy. Best known for the foundational documents of the profession on nursing ethics, scope and standards of practice, and social policy, Nursesbooks.org is the publisher for the professional, career-oriented nurse, reaching and serving nurse educators, administrators, managers, and researchers, as well as staff nurses in the course of their professional development.

# The Need for Safe Patient Handling and Mobility (SPHM) Standards

Healthcare workers continue to be needlessly injured on the job. During 2011, workers in the healthcare/social assistance sector suffered a higher rate of musculoskeletal disorders (MSDs) than construction, mining, or manufacturing workers (Figure 1; BLS, 2012).

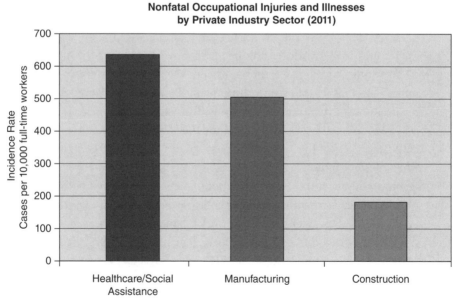

**Figure 1.** 2011 Nonfatal Occupational Injuries and Illness by Private Industry Sector

**Source:** Bureau of Labor Statistics, U.S Department of Labor, October 2012

According to ANA's 2011 health and safety survey, 62% of registered nurses indicated that suffering a disabling MSD was one of their top three safety concerns, and 80% reported working despite experiencing frequent musculoskeletal pain (ANA, 2011). In 2011, registered nurses ranked fifth among all occupations for the number of cases of musculoskeletal disorders resulting in days away from work, with 11,880 total cases. Nursing assistants reported 25,010 cases, the highest for any occupation. These injuries were serious enough to result in lost work time (BLS, 2012).

The majority of injuries and MSDs can be attributed to overexertion related to repeated transfer, repositioning, and ambulation of healthcare recipients (OSHA, 2011). Societal trends, such as an aging population and increasing obesity of both healthcare recipients and healthcare workers, have aggravated the problem. Healthcare provision is also more complex, as services are delivered across a broader continuum of care.

Safe patient handling and mobility (SPHM) programs, if properly implemented, can drastically reduce healthcare worker injuries. Many healthcare organizations have SPHM policies, but have encountered challenges in implementing and sustaining programs. At the time this document was published, only 10 states had enacted laws related to the implementation of SPHM programs, and the SPHM program components mandated within those laws are not consistent.

Universal SPHM standards are needed to protect healthcare workers from injuries and MSDs. Addressing healthcare worker safety through SPHM will also improve the safety of healthcare recipients (patients). The Joint Commission (TJC) monograph, "Improving Patient and Worker Safety," and the Lucian Leape Institute's "Through the Eyes of the Workforce" were recently published. Both publications demonstrate the increased recognition and intent to raise awareness of the intersection between healthcare worker and healthcare recipient safety, indicating that safer environments of care increase quality of patient care (TJC, 2012; National Patient Safety Foundation [NPSF], 2013).

Stakeholders across the continuum of care are promoting the implementation of SPHM to protect healthcare workers and healthcare recipients. Each profession brings a different perspective, goal, and terminology. ANA recognized the need for a universal set of SPHM standards that can be applied to all healthcare settings and used by all healthcare workers across the continuum of care.

# Development of the SPHM Standards

The standard development process was designed to maximize collaboration across professions for the benefit of the healthcare recipient. Figure 2 illustrates the steps of the process.

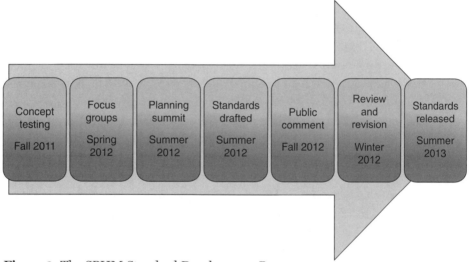

**Figure 2.** The SPHM Standard Development Process

## Concept Testing

The concepts of universal standards and an interdisciplinary approach to care emerged from resources developed by the Centers for Medicare and Medicaid Services (CMS), the Institute of Medicine (IOM), the World Health Organization (WHO), and the National Quality Foundation (NQF) (CMS, 2013; IOM, 2012; WHO, 2010; NQF, 2013). Additionally, the need for universal SPHM standards was supported by results from the American Nurses Association's 2011 Health and Safety Survey. The survey indicated that patient

handling and lifting injuries remain a topic of concern, despite many education and legislative efforts.

ANA presented the need for universal SPHM standards at the 11th Annual
Safe Patient Handling East Conference in March 2011. The concept was very
well received.

## Focus Groups

Focus groups were assembled during the 12th Annual Safe Patient Handling
East Conference in Orlando (March 2012), to explore the need for universal
standards and to begin to compile a list of the subject matter experts, professional organizations, industry groups, and government agencies to involve.
Planning activities identified the need for an interprofessional summit to bring
these individuals together and begin discussions.

## Formation of the Work Group and National Summit

The Work Group was comprised of national subject-matter experts identified
from across multiple healthcare disciplines. Representatives were included
from nursing, physical and occupational therapy, public health, loss control,
ergonomics, and long-term care. Work Group members were professionals
employed in direct patient care and/or healthcare management; members and
staff of professional associations; consultants; and representatives from the
federal government, including the U.S. Department of Veterans Affairs, the U.S.
Army, and the National Institute of Occupational Safety and Health (NIOSH).

ANA's Department for Health, Safety, and Wellness hosted a summit on
June 29, 2012, at ANA's headquarters in Silver Spring, Maryland, to dis-
cuss a framework for the universal standards. Members of the Work Group
were invited to attend. Most attended in person; several attended virtually.
Participants traveling to the summit paid their own expenses.

Technology and insurance vendors participated to share their expertise in
implementation of SPHM programs across a variety of healthcare settings.
However, ANA funded the development and publication of the standards; no
external funding was offered or accepted.

## Setting the Foundation

Prior to the summit, ANA staff conducted a comprehensive literature review
and provided the Work Group with key documents and publications related

to SPHM (Appendix B). ANA staff also identified expectations for the SPHM standards and presented them to the Work Group at the summit. The SPHM standards were expected to be:

- Useful in healthcare settings across the continuum of care

- Useful for healthcare workers, ancillary/support staff, and organizational leadership

- Realistic and attainable, while raising the bar

- Evidence-based and outcome-focused

During the summit, the Work Group reviewed and agreed on the expectations. In addition, the Work Group was reminded that standards are to be overarching and are not to be prescriptive, allowing organizations and employers to decide on the best way to implement the standards for their particular situations.

The Work Group determined that the SPHM standards must clearly define the roles and responsibilities of employers and healthcare workers, recognizing that successful implementation of SPHM programs requires the commitment of both groups.

The Work Group next prioritized what was to be included in the universal standards, identified important healthcare trends, and began to identify and develop a common terminology. To address the evidence-based trend toward progressive mobility as a healthcare recipient goal, "and Mobility" was added to the title "Safe Patient Handling." The Work Group identified 10 content areas to be included in the SPHM standards and formed sub-groups to develop each content area.

## SPHM Standards Drafted

Drafts of the standards, definitions, and interpretive language were developed by each of the sub-groups over an intensive eight-week period during late summer 2012. A technical writer with subject-matter expertise, ANA staff, and the Work Group chair reviewed the documents for repetition and distilled the writings down to eight distinct standards. The eight standards were returned to the Work Group for editing and revision during the fall of 2012. The Work Group used a consensus process to establish concepts and definitions that held more than one meaning for members of different professions or healthcare settings.

## Public Comment

The public was invited to comment on the draft standards during the fall of 2012. Responses were received from 234 individuals, professional organizations, healthcare organizations, vendors, and government agencies. More than 500 distinct comments were provided. Public comments focused on existing barriers to SPHM, identified concerns related to the work environment, and affirmed the need for universal standards.

Standards 1.1.2 Nonpunitive Environment, 1.1.3 Right of Refusal, and 1.1.4 Safe Staffing drew intense, emotional responses during the public comment period. Reviewers from a variety of professions and healthcare settings reported feeling afraid to report errors, refuse an unsafe care assignment, or report unsafe staffing.

Public reviewers were sensitive to the cost of SPHM technology and supplies, and recommended that organizations establish priorities, and develop a plan and timeline for procurement. Healthcare workers in the community setting wrote about the persistent lack of SPHM technology during the first few home health visits, and the resulting risk to healthcare workers, as well as healthcare recipients and their families. The reviewers believed that poor discharge planning related to SPHM technology could lead to injuries and unnecessary hospitalizations. These concerns informed the development of Standard 6.1.4 on transitions of care.

The public reviewers focused on needing sufficient time to learn about SPHM, and on being short-staffed when healthcare workers were away at training. Standards 1.1.4, on safe staffing, and 5.1.3, on providing time for education and training, were included to address the need for budgeting for staff development.

Standard 6.1.5, requiring a system to address the healthcare recipient's right of refusal, drew attention. One reviewer wrote, "How can a patient require that I lift manually when I know that I will be hurt? Shouldn't safety for both of us be a condition of care?" The Work Group discussed the importance of having a formal system for addressing healthcare recipient refusal of SPHM technology.

## Review and Revisions

Public comments were considered and incorporated as appropriate. Through a collaborative and collegial effort, the Work Group, ANA staff, and the technical writer again reviewed and revised the standards during the winter of 2013. The standards were also reviewed by the ANA Committee on Nursing Practice Standards.

# Trends and Issues Influencing the Development of the SPHM Standards

The following section summarizes the research, historical context, health considerations, and environment-of-care factors that influenced the development of the SPHM standards. The SPHM standards are written with the understanding that manual handling is hazardous and that a comprehensive SPHM program, which includes appropriate technology, is necessary for lifting, moving, and mobilizing the dependent healthcare recipient.

## A Paradigm Shift to Safety: The Elimination of Manual Handling

Musculoskeletal disorders and injuries associated with patient handling and mobility have been a healthcare risk for many years. Nurses have often been blamed for their own injuries, as illustrated in this quote from *Nursing: Its Principles and Practices*, the first major nursing textbook: "Occasionally the complaint is made that a nurse has injured her back or strained herself in some way in moving a patient. This will generally be because she has failed to do the lifting properly" (Hampton, 1898).

More than a hundred years later, in 2003, ANA released a position statement titled "The Elimination of Manual Patient Handling to Prevent Work-Related Musculoskeletal Disorders." Within that document, ANA asserted that "manual patient handling is unsafe and is directly responsible for musculoskeletal disorders suffered by nurses." Updated in 2008, ANA supported establishment of a safe environment of care for nurses and patients through actions and policies that result in the elimination of manual patient handling

(ANA, 2008). In conjunction with the release of the position statement, ANA launched its Handle with Care© campaign as an industry-wide initiative to prevent back and musculoskeletal disorders and injuries for both patients and the nursing workforce (ANA, 2012a).

This paradigm shift within nursing was based on a large body of research demonstrating that "lifting properly"—that is, using good body mechanics—cannot protect nurses or other healthcare workers (Waters, 2007; Nelson, Fragala, & Menzel, 2003). Based on available evidence, manual handling is unsafe in almost every situation. SPHM technology and methods must be used to lift, laterally transfer, or reposition dependent healthcare recipients.

## Demographics and Characteristics of the U.S. Healthcare Population

The U.S. population is aging. The proportion of Americans 65 years of age and older is expected to increase from 12% in 2005 to approximately 20% by 2030. This will have a major impact on how health care is organized and delivered in all environments of care. An aging population will result in a shift from acute care to the chronic management of multiple illnesses and disabilities (Wiener & Tilly, 2002; IOM, 2008). As a result, more Americans will depend on care in community settings, including long-term care and in the home.

Obesity is highly prevalent among adults in the U.S. population. During 2010, 33.3% of the United States adult population was considered overweight, and another 35.9% was considered obese. Approximately 6.9% are considered extremely obese (Fryar, Carroll, & Ogden, 2012). These statistics apply to both healthcare recipients and healthcare workers.

Due to the increasing weight of healthcare recipients, and the recognition that obese and morbidly obese healthcare recipients are at particularly high risk for complications of immobility, new technologies are being developed. Organizations have developed policies and procedures, and designated bariatric beds or units with special technology to meet the unique needs of this population.

Despite advances in accommodating healthcare recipients, factors such as age and obesity are stressors on the healthcare delivery system. As a result, hospital stays have shortened and healthcare recipients receive care in community settings at an earlier stage of recovery. This increases dependency on healthcare workers in community settings and exposes both healthcare workers and healthcare recipients to greater risk of injury (National Center for Health Statistics [NCHS], 2010; NIOSH, 2010).

## Healthcare Recipient vs. Patient

Describing the "patient" was a challenge, as the standards are intended to be used interprofessionally, in a variety of settings and environments of care, across the continuum of care. Persons receiving care are identified differently by healthcare professions within different environments of care. Hospitals and clinics have *in-patients* and *out-patients*. In long-term care, the preferred terminology is *resident*. Those working in mental health and insurance settings address *consumers* or *persons*; ambulatory care has *clients*; and schools have *students*. Such variation of terms can make it difficult to communicate.

For the purposes of this document, the Work Group decided that the term *healthcare recipient* is more inclusive and will be used, except when describing research where the term "patient" was used, and in terminology where the term "patient" is currently ingrained, such as in the name of "safe patient handling" or "patient-centered care."

The Work Group recognized the importance of interprofessional dialogue and including the healthcare recipient and family caregivers in the development of a SPHM component of the plan of care. Therefore, within the standards, patient families and volunteer caregivers are included within the definition of *healthcare recipient*.

## The Interprofessional Healthcare Team

The interprofessional nature of the SPHM standards is emphasized throughout the document. These standards are intended as a guide for multiple professionals in diverse settings. Organizational leaders and practitioners will need to translate how the standards apply to their specific settings.

The Work Group wanted an inclusive term for the many people who provide direct care, including, but not limited to: nurses, therapists, physicians, paramedics, technicians, technologists, aides, unlicensed assistive personnel, and others. The term *healthcare worker* is used throughout these standards, except when citing research that identifies a specific professional.

The Work Group recognized that a SPHM program is impossible without ancillary and support staff. Within these standards, the term *ancillary/support staff* is defined to include staff members from departments such as consultants, risk management, safety, infection prevention, occupational health, transportation, security, activity direction, recreational therapy, creative art therapy, environmental services, laundry, volunteers, engineering, biomedical engineering, facilities, morgue, funeral home, purchasing, and contracting.

The term *organizational leadership* is used to identify those individuals who establish objectives, plans, and policies and allocate the resources within a place or employment organization. The term managers includes mid-level persons who ensure that plans and policies are carried out to meet the organizational objectives. Within these standards, the term *organizational leadership* is inclusive of managers.

## Continuum of Care

Today, patient handling and mobility occurs in many different environments of care, and each has unique hazards, challenges, and opportunities. The Work Group considered pre-acute care, hospital units, bariatrics, surgery, rehabilitation, long-term care, assisted living, home care, hospice, ambulatory care, occupational health, group homes, schools, correctional facilities, morgues, and other settings. Standard 6 addresses the individual healthcare recipient within the continuum of care. The standards also contain considerations for nonhospital or community settings.

The Work Group observed that SPHM is particularly difficult at transitions of care. Prehospital emergency care is particularly hazardous, as the environment may prevent the healthcare worker from using SPHM technology to transfer healthcare recipients across barriers, up or down steps, out of bed, or off the floor or ground. Dependent or combative healthcare recipients may need to be transferred quickly across slippery or uneven surfaces, at night and in conditions with poor visibility.

Transitions within environments of care can also be difficult to manage. SPHM documentation may or may not be included in a shift report or health record. The healthcare recipient's specific SPHM technology needs may be present in one environment of care, but not available in others, such as emergency department, radiology, therapy, or long-term care.

Healthcare recipients being discharged from acute or long-term care require a designed plan that considers their living environment. The home environment may have steps, carpet, narrow doorways, small bathrooms, and low couches or beds. The appropriate SPHM technology must be in place when the healthcare recipient arrives at the next care setting, and the healthcare worker and/or caregiver must have instruction and be comfortable with using that technology.

Finally, the healthcare recipient is typically responsible for payment in the home setting, and may be unable to afford appropriate SPHM technology. Local medical supply vendors may not have up-to-date SPHM technology or the specific technology that provides therapeutic value to an individual healthcare recipient. The healthcare recipient may need to travel to medical or therapy appointments, to congregant care, or to school. The plan of care should address activities of daily living, like toileting and bathing, as well as transportation.

## Culture of Safety

The concept of a culture of safety evolved from studies of high-reliability industries outside of health care. Individuals working in these areas, such as air traffic controllers and nuclear power plant employees, do complex and hazardous work, while maintaining a commitment to safety at all times. Key features of a culture of safety include acknowledgment of the risk, a commitment to provide resources to consistently achieve safe operations, a blame-free environment where individuals are able to report errors or incidents without fear, and an emphasis on collaboration across sectors and settings (Pizzi, Goldfarb, & Nash, 2001).

A culture of safety in health care encompasses the core values and behaviors resulting from a collective, consistent, and sustained commitment by organizational leadership, managers, healthcare workers, and ancillary/support staff to emphasize safety over competing goals. Leaders drive the culture of safety by demonstrating their own commitment; providing the resources to achieve the desired results; and ensuring that policies, themes, and behaviors related to safety become widely accepted practice. A culture of safety in health care includes a fair and nonpunitive culture, as described in "Just Culture" principles; a process for right of refusal; a system for safe staffing; and open, collaborative, and congenial communication.

The concept of a fair and "Just Culture" evolved from the work of behavioral, management, and clinical researchers who found that the way an organization responds to errors influences the prevention of future errors. An organization that practices "Just Culture" recognizes that many errors are caused by predictable interactions between employees and the systems they work in. Competent employees do make errors and must be encouraged to report those errors. This information is used by the organization to investigate causes and to correct system issues. Employees (e.g., the healthcare workers) are not held responsible for system issues over which they have no control, but are held accountable for reckless behavior (ANA, 2010; Frankel, Leonard, & Denham, 2006).

Specific to nursing, it is the ethical responsibility of every registered nurse to protect the health and safety of patients and self. The ANA position statement, *Patient Safety: Rights of Registered Nurses When Considering a Patient*

*Assignment,* addresses the concept of right of refusal (ANA, 2009). The position statement lists recommendations for registered nurses, the employer/healthcare agency, and the patient and consumer. The statement distinguishes between refusing an assignment before accepting responsibility and abandoning the care of a patient.

The 2012 *ANA's Principles for Nurse Staffing* identifies the major elements needed to achieve optimal staffing, which enhances the delivery of safe, quality care. The principles and supporting material in that publication guide nurses and other decision-makers in identifying and developing the processes and policies needed to improve nurse staffing at every practice level and in any practice setting (ANA, 2012b).

Communication and collaboration are critical to establishing a culture of safety and to the success of a SPHM program. The organization is charged with developing or utilizing a variety of communication systems to inform and engage the healthcare worker. Collaboration among leaders, managers, healthcare workers, ancillary/support staff, and healthcare recipients was consolidated into Standard 1.1.5 for simplicity and clarity. The Work Group also considered the importance of clear and consistent communication and collaboration within and between specific settings and environments of care.

## Use of SPHM to Promote Mobility and Improve Safety

The benefits of early mobilization and the hazards of immobility are well documented in the literature. Research demonstrating the relationship between SPHM and healthcare recipient outcomes is limited, but encouraging. For example, Nelson et al. described the link between safe patient handling and patient outcomes in long-term care (Nelson, Collins, Siddarthan, Matz, & Waters, 2008). Following implementation of a six-point SPHM program, patients exhibited lower levels of depression, improved urinary continence, higher alertness and engagement in activities of daily living, and decreased fall risk, pain, and combativeness.

Researchers from South Africa described the importance of early, progressive mobilization for critically ill patients and commented that removal of barriers facilitates the use of mobility as a powerful intervention to reduce respiratory complications and ICU-acquired weakness (Hannekom, 2011).

The term *safe patient handling and movement* has been used since the 1980s to describe formal efforts to handle and move healthcare recipients. *Movement* implies a passive state, describing the healthcare worker moving the healthcare recipient. The term *mobility* was selected to imply the involvement of the healthcare recipient and the potential for improved outcomes. This is consistent with the evidence-based trend of using SPHM technology to promote early mobilization in the acute care setting, and with rehabilitation efforts in long-term care that have the goal of rehabilitation and restoration of independence, as appropriate.

New technologies promote healthcare recipient independence through earlier mobility and ambulation, safer transfers to chair or toilet, and technologies to assist with activities of daily living. Standard 6 recognizes that SPHM technology incorporates more than assistive lifting equipment, and thus focuses on the provision of care to individuals and facilitation of the use of a variety of SPHM technologies as therapeutic modalities for promoting independence. Though often not thought of as SPHM technology, the electronic health record should be used as a tool to promote communication and follow through across the continuum of care.

## Safe Lifting Limits

One of the goals of SPHM is to identify high-risk tasks for healthcare workers, and minimize the impact of risk factors such as force, repetition, and posture. The "Revised NIOSH Lifting Equation" provides documentation for the recommendation that no worker should lift more than 51 pounds and notes that the calculations do not apply to healthcare workers because these workers do not lift stable loads, loads with handles, or loads that can be held close to the body (Waters, Putz-Anderson, & Garg, 1994).

Evidence is available to provide guidance regarding the use of interventions such as SPHM technology. Considering the "Revised NIOSH Lifting Equation," Waters has proposed that when weight exceeds 35 pounds, assistive devices should be used (Waters, 2007; Waters, Putz-Anderson, & Garg, 1994). The 35-pound limit should be further reduced if the healthcare worker is lifting in a restricted space, while sitting or kneeling, near the floor, twisting, one-handed, or with arms extended. The 35-pound limit should also be reduced if the healthcare worker is working longer than an eight-hour shift, or if the healthcare recipient is combative, cannot follow directions, or has physical or medical conditions that impact his or her being lifted or moved (Waters, 2007).

Pushing and pulling motions, required repositioning, and lateral transfers of healthcare recipients also put healthcare workers at risk of injury. Additional sources provide evidence to suggest guidelines for limits to determine when SPHM technology should be applied to reduce risks related to these activities (Snook, 1991).

It is a common misconception that healthcare workers who are strong or physically fit can safely lift healthcare recipients manually. Conversely, research has shown that worker physical fitness may *increase* the exposure to risk of injury. The Veterans Health Administration Technical Advisory Group reported that physically fit healthcare workers are asked to help four times more often, and thus are exposed to more risk (VISN 8, 2005).

## Evolution of SPHM Technology

The original lift equipment used in health care was adapted from other industries and was based on the movement of static loads, such as boxes. This early equipment caused some discomfort for healthcare recipients and had limited adaptability to a range of activities or healthcare settings.

Researchers and vendors responded by conceptualizing and developing a wide variety of new SPHM technology to assist with lifting, repositioning, lateral transfers, sit to stand, toileting, bathing, ambulation, and travel. SPHM technology has been developed to meet the needs of specific environments of care, such as emergency response and home care, as well as specific healthcare recipient populations, including bariatric patients, children, and people with amputations.

SPHM technology may include, but is not limited to: equipment for moving, lifting, transferring, stand assist, and ambulation; bathing equipment; ceiling lifts; commode/shower chairs; lateral transfer equipment or mattresses; portable lifts, slides, or slide boards; repositioning equipment; specialty beds and mattresses; transfer chairs and cushions; and wheelchairs and stretchers. The term *technology* is used to recognize that support means more than lifting and mobilizing equipment, also including accessories, software, and multimedia resources used for education and evaluative monitoring.

SPHM technology must be accessible to be used, so an adequate amount must be procured and conveniently stored. The Work Group recommends the use of ergonomic evaluation methods specific to the healthcare recipient for the appropriate environment of care. Subject-matter experts can determine the types and quantity of SPHM technology needed, based on the unique physical layout and healthcare recipient population of each environment of care. NIOSH estimates that the ideal number is approximately one full lift for every eight to ten non-weight-bearing residents and approximately one sit-to-stand lift for every eight to ten partially weight-bearing residents (Collins, 2006).

## Barriers to SPHM Technology Use

The National Council on Compensation Insurance (NCCI), in collaboration with the University of Maryland, conducted a national study of long-term care facilities that had safe-lifting programs. The initial intent of the study was to compare facilities with and without programs, but the results indicated that by the end of the study period, nearly 95% of facilities had SPHM technology and close to 80% routinely used it. Therefore, the NCCI concluded that the real question was whether the organizations had implemented a comprehensive safe patient handling program. Important variables were the existence and enforcement of policies and procedures, training and preferences of the Director of Nursing, and the perception of barriers (Restrepo, 2013).

Common barriers to use include inadequate quantities of SPHM technology, or technology that is difficult to use, incompatible, or improperly cleaned or maintained. Access to SPHM technology is another major barrier. Access issues may result when SPHM technology is located in an inconvenient place or difficult to use due to space restraints (Nelson & Fragala, 2004).

Environments of care must be carefully designed to facilitate access to and use of SPHM technology. NIOSH, in collaboration with the American Industrial Hygiene Association (AIHA), the American Society of Safety Engineers (ASSE), the Center to Protect Workers' Rights, Kaiser Permanente, Liberty Mutual, the National Safety Council (NSC), the Occupational Safety and Health Administration (OSHA), ORC Worldwide, and the Regenstrief Center for Healthcare Engineering developed the national initiative called Prevention through Design (PtD) (ANSI/ASSE, 2011). Ergonomic design principles such as PtD must be addressed during every remodeling or construction project on healthcare recipient environments of care. Examples include building or retrofitting ceilings to support ceiling lifts, wide doorways, adequate space to maneuver, portable lifts in healthcare recipient bathrooms, and the installation of flooring that facilitates smooth movement of wheeled heavy loads.

Seeking input related to perceived barriers can increase healthcare worker engagement in SPHM. Research demonstrates that barriers to use can effectively be resolved if addressed prior to implementation of SPHM programs (Wardell, 2007). It is also essential for organizational leadership to continually reinforce that SPHM is an expectation of care.

## Learning Healthcare Systems

The IOM report on the Continuous Learning Healthcare System describes strategies to generate and apply the best evidence for the collaborative healthcare choices of each healthcare recipient and provider. The report encourages the use of computing power, connectivity, team-based care, and systems engineering techniques. A learning healthcare system aligns science and informatics, patient clinician partnerships, incentives, and a culture of continuous improvement to produce the best care at lower cost (IOM, 2012). Algorithms or scoring systems within the electronic health record will support selection of appropriate SPHM technology and methods to benefit the healthcare recipient across the continuum of care. A fully integrated system would facilitate reports to help evaluate the effectiveness of the SPHM intervention and/or program.

Until a learning healthcare system is in place, stakeholders and organizational leaders need to collect various data and conduct a careful evaluation of the SPHM program. Standard 8 and Appendix A suggest data and information sources for formative and summative evaluation.

## Quality and Safety Measures

Healthcare quality and safety have received intense focus since the 1999 Institute of Medicine report, *To Err Is Human: Building a Safer Health System* (IOM, 2000). The Patient Safety and Quality Improvement Act of 2005 encourages healthcare organizations to voluntarily measure and track adverse events and reduce the barriers to care improvement by encouraging voluntary organizational change and sharing of data.

The National Quality Strategy is designed to increase access to high-quality, affordable health care for all Americans. Healthcare organizations and providers are challenged to reduce healthcare-related injury to an incidence of zero. Standard 6.1.6 requires the organization to monitor injuries associated with patient handling and mobility.

There are multiple national initiatives aimed at improving healthcare recipient safety and outcomes. The Partnership for Patients, a program of the Centers for Medicare and Medicaid Innovation, has targeted the end of 2013 for decreasing preventable hospital-acquired conditions by 40%, as compared with 2010. Achieving this goal would mean approximately 1.8 million fewer injuries to healthcare recipients, with more than 60,000 lives saved over 3 years (Agency for Healthcare Research and Quality [AHRQ], 2012).

The American Nurses Association launched its Patient Safety and Quality Initiative in 1994 and subsequently developed the National Database of Nursing Quality Indicators® (NDNQI®) as a result. The purpose of the NDNQI is to collect and build upon existing data and further develop the body of knowledge related to the factors that influence the quality of care (Montalvo, 2007).

Healthcare organizations are using the NDNQI® to identify the structure and processes that improve safety and outcomes of care. A SPHM program may impact a variety of NDNQI measures, including pressure ulcers. For instance, Sturman-Floyd found strong evidence that ceiling lift systems can reduce pressure ulcer incidence, and are particularly useful for home care patients who are bariatric, frail, have tissue viability problems, or express physically challenging behaviors. She noted that fewer staff were needed to move the patients, and that by using the equipment, family members could turn and reposition the patients between professional care visits (Sturman-Floyd, 2012). Other NDNQI® measures related to SPHM may include (but are not limited to) falls with injury, restraints, and decubitus ulcer.

## SPHM Funding

Healthcare organizations are under increasing financial pressure and uncertainty as regulations governing the Affordable Care Act are developed and implemented. An analysis of return on investment (ROI) will demonstrate the value of investing in a comprehensive SPHM program. New, sophisticated models provide a range of savings for both direct costs (medical and lost time, worker's compensation, replacement of healthcare workers, Medicare penalties for falls and pressure ulcers) and indirect costs (management time, turnover, and patient and staff satisfaction) (Facilities Guidelines Institute [FGI], 2010b).

Changes in healthcare financing have resulted in more complex care being delivered within the community. The Work Group acknowledges the need for insurance and other third-party payers to consistently provide payment for appropriate SPHM technology in the community, as indicated in the individual plan of care. For example, adults with physical impairments may need several technologies to enable full mobility at home. Children with disabilities who attend school may need SPHM technology at home and at school. The Work Group recommends that healthcare recipient and provider associations advocate for access to SPHM technology for their unique populations.

## Return to Work

Historically, patient handling and mobility has been dependent on the ability of people to manually lift and move other people. This required a certain level of physical ability that had the effect of excluding some healthcare workers from employment in direct patient care. These facts have changed, as SPHM programs now use methods and technologies to minimize the risk of patient handling and mobility.

Standard 7 addresses the disabled and injured healthcare worker. Various laws, such as the Americans with Disabilities Act and state-based worker's compensation laws, may apply to disabled and injured healthcare workers. It is not the purpose of these voluntary standards to rewrite law, but instead to encourage the use of SPHM programs as an evidence-based strategy for meeting the intent of these laws.

## Legal Requirements for Safe Patient Handling and Mobility

A legal framework supporting adoption and implementation of a SPHM program does exist. The "General Duty Clause" of the United States Occupational Safety and Health Act, 29 U.S.C. § 654, 5(a)1 (federal OSHA), states that "[e]ach employer shall furnish to each of his employees, employment and a place of employment which are free from recognized hazards that are causing or are likely to cause death or serious physical harm to his employees." State laws impose similar duties and require employers to mitigate hazards and risks. As these standards go to press, laws related to safe patient handling are on the books in 10 states (Figure 3). The standards in *Safe Patient Handling and Mobility: Interprofessional National Standards* are designed to be incorporated into practice, policy, procedure, law, and regulation.

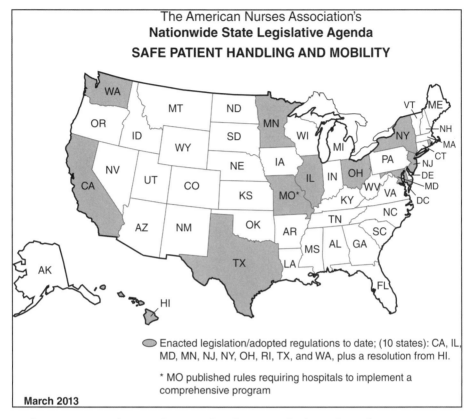

**Figure 3.** Map of enacted SPHM legislation and adopted regulations.

**Source:** ANA, 2013. nursingworld.org/MainMenuCategories/Policy-Advocacy/
State/Legislative-Agenda-Reports/State-SafePatientHandling

# Organization and Intent of the SPHM Standards

This document contains eight overarching SPHM standards of care, each of which is organized into two parts: (1) standards addressing the responsibilities of the employer or healthcare organization, and (2) standards addressing the responsibilities of the healthcare worker and ancillary/support staff, with descriptive comments accompanying each.

Special considerations for community settings are included to address current differences. The vignettes (explained on the next page and featured as sidebars of each standard's opening page) are fictional examples of situations experienced by healthcare workers and healthcare recipients, and are meant to illustrate and clarify the intent and implementation of specific standards.

This document is designed to be used by many different professionals across the care continuum. The document is intended to be used across healthcare settings and adapted by the user to specific settings, whenever possible.

The Work Group envisions that healthcare organizations may adopt these standards to improve the quality and safety of care, and prevent injuries among healthcare workers and healthcare recipients. Insurance companies and other third-party payers may adopt these SPHM standards as an indication of quality and a condition of payment. Regulatory agencies may adopt or adapt these standards to control or improve the services of an industry. The SPHM standards may be used by the legal profession as evidence of the standard of care and to inform regulatory decisions.

---

*Note: The SPHM standards are open, voluntary standards. The standards do not require use of any specific products or services. ANA and the endorsing organizations do not promote, endorse, or recommend any products or services.*

---

The American Nurses Association and stakeholder contributors recognize that change takes time and resources, and recommend that organizations perform a needs assessment; establish priorities, goals, and objectives; develop a timeline for implementation and evaluation; and use the SPHM standards to create a safe environment of care.

### SPHM Standards in Daily Practice

Throughout the following section, for each of the eight SPHM standards you will find a vignette—an example scenario showing how that standard might prove useful in overcoming some familiar barriers to SPHM encountered in daily practice. Each vignette (as shown in the example below) also identifies other standards that might also come into play.

These standards address the core issues, and will guide healthcare organizations to provide a safer work environment and improved patient outcomes.

---

**IN DAILY PRACTICE ...**

MELANIE IS A MANAGER ON A MEDICAL–SURGICAL UNIT. "We are in the old part of the hospital and are the last to get new stuff. It always goes to the ICUs and the newer units first. I am working with risk management to evaluate the preventable injuries and maybe make a case for some SPHM technology. I think it would help with retention of staff, too. I really care about my staff and our patients, but body mechanics alone just doesn't cut it. I just wonder how many people will get hurt before things change."

*(See also Standards 1, 2, 3, 5, and 8.)*

---

# Interprofessional Standards of Safe Patient Handling and Mobility

## Standard 1. Establish a Culture of Safety

The employer and healthcare workers partner to establish a culture of safety that encompasses the core values and behaviors resulting from a collective and sustained commitment by organizational leadership, managers, healthcare workers, and ancillary/support staff to emphasize safety over competing goals.

### 1.1 EMPLOYER

**1.1.1 Establish a statement of commitment to a culture of safety**
Organizational policy will include a written commitment to a culture of safety that will be used to guide the organization's priorities, resource allocation, policies, and procedures. The written statement regarding SPHM will describe layers of accountability across sectors and settings.

**IN DAILY PRACTICE ...**

ARUN, A **46**-YEAR-OLD SURGICAL TECH, remembers the last hospital he worked in. "We had a really cool air mattress to move patients from the gurney to the surgery table and back, and special equipment for the heaviest people. Here, we use a draw sheet and get three or four or five or six of us to work together. It's hard on my back, but it is even harder on the patient's skin. We are all afraid to say something, because the hospital is short of money and we don't want to get fired for complaining."

*(See also Standards 2, 4, 6, and 8.)*

---

*NOTE: The SPHM standards are open, voluntary standards. The standards do not require use of any specific products or services. ANA and the endorsing organizations do not promote, endorse, or recommend any products or services.*

---

### 1.1.2 Establish a nonpunitive environment

Organizational policy will support a system to encourage healthcare workers to report hazards, errors, incidents, and accidents, so that the precursors to SPHM errors can be better understood and organizational issues can be changed to prevent future incidents and injuries. Healthcare workers know that they are accountable for their actions, but will not be held accountable for problems within the system or environment that are beyond their control.

### 1.1.3 Provide a system for right of refusal

Organizational policy will provide the healthcare worker the right to accept, reject, or object to any healthcare recipient transfer, repositioning, or mobility assignment that puts the healthcare recipient or the healthcare worker at risk for injury. The refusal shall be made in writing, without fear of retribution. The policy will describe steps for resolving the hazard.

### 1.1.4 Provide safe levels of staffing

An evidence-based system will be used to determine safe and appropriate case-loads. Adequate staffing levels will support safe patient handling and mobility, including allocated time for training and education.

### 1.1.5 Establish a system for communication and collaboration

Collaboration among all sectors and settings is critical. The organization will utilize a variety of communication systems to inform and engage the healthcare workers and healthcare recipients about SPHM.

## 1.2 HEALTHCARE WORKER

### 1.2.1 Participate in creating and maintaining a culture of safety

The healthcare worker will actively participate in creating and maintaining a culture of safety.

### 1.2.2 Notify the employer of hazards, incidents, near misses, and accidents

The healthcare worker will notify the employer of hazards, near misses, incidents, and accidents related to SPHM as soon as possible, using the reporting procedures defined by the employer.

### 1.2.3 Use the system to communicate and collaborate

The healthcare worker will engage, verbally and in writing, with others about SPHM.

**CONSIDERATIONS FOR COMMUNITY SETTINGS**

The community setting provides unique challenges for the correction of hazards. For example, in home health, the healthcare worker is a guest in the home, and the healthcare recipient is typically financially responsible for the environment of care. Hazardous conditions, broken or inappropriate technology, or unreasonable requests must be discussed with the healthcare recipient and reported to the employer. The employer is ultimately responsible for the health of employees and can determine if engineering or other controls are available to correct the hazards, or determine that care cannot be safely provided.

## Standard 2. Implement and Sustain a Safe Patient Handling and Mobility (SPHM) Program

The employer and healthcare workers partner to establish a formal, systematized SPHM program for reducing the risk of injury to healthcare recipients and the risk of injuries and MSDs in healthcare workers, while improving the quality of care.

### 2.1 EMPLOYER

**2.1.1 Designate a group or groups of stakeholders to develop, implement, evaluate, remediate, and maintain a SPHM program**

An organizational committee will identify or develop systems that support SPHM programs. The committee will receive and review data about SPHM and make recommendations for improvement. The work of the committee will reflect collaboration among organizational leadership, the healthcare worker, and ancillary/support workers.

> **IN DAILY PRACTICE ...**
>
> JAY, A 27-YEAR-OLD RN, enjoys his work in the pediatric ICU. "I worry about my back. Most of our patients aren't really large, but we are bending and reaching a lot. I get called to lift when the patients' parents code, seize, or have a low blood sugar. I guess they think that because I am a guy, I can lift more! A few days ago, a large man fell in the bathroom and no one knew how to get him up off the floor. A children's hospital just doesn't have that kind of equipment. . . ."
>
> *(See also Standards 1, 4, 5, and 8.)*

**2.1.2 Perform a comprehensive assessment of SPHM**

The organization will initially and periodically perform a comprehensive assessment of patient handling, mobility, and technology, including a SPHM technology needs assessment (see Standard 4.1.1).

**2.1.3 Develop a written SPHM program, with goals, objectives, and a plan for ongoing evaluation, compliance, and quality improvement**

The written SPHM program will address each of the eight standards of *Safe Patient Handling and Mobility: Interprofessional National Standards*, and will reflect compliance with federal, state, and local laws and regulations. The written program will include short- and long-term goals and objectives, and a realistic plan and timeline to meet the goals and evaluation requirements. The written SPHM program will identify, by title, those individuals who have responsibility, authority, and accountability for developing and implementing the plan. The written SPHM program also will establish a clear reporting hierarchy to monitor compliance.

**2.1.4 Customize and integrate the SPHM program across the continuum of care**
The SPHM program will be customized for, and integrated into, care settings throughout the organization and continuum of care, ensuring that SPHM is addressed through transitions of care.

**2.1.5 Provide funding to implement and sustain the program**
The employer will identify and allocate funding to implement and sustain the program based on business-case and return-on-investment analytics or cost/benefit analysis.

**2.1.6 Identify the essential physical functions and high-risk tasks of jobs**
The organization will identify the essential physical functions of a job in a written job description. An evidence-based process or review of scientific literature will be used to identify activities that place the healthcare worker at high risk for injury.

**2.1.7 Reduce the physical requirements of high-risk tasks**
The organization will focus on reducing the physical requirements of high-risk healthcare recipient transfer, repositioning, and mobilization, and other applicable tasks through engineering, safe work practice, and/or administrative controls.

**2.2 HEALTHCARE WORKERS**

**2.2.1 Participate in the SPHM program**
The healthcare worker will actively engage in the SPHM program, following the policies and procedures of the organization's SPHM program.

**CONSIDERATIONS FOR COMMUNITY SETTINGS**
The healthcare recipient is financially responsible for procurement of SPHM technology in most home, community, and school settings. The coordination of care at transition from acute or long-term care settings must address mobility needs. The organization and/or healthcare worker can assist by identifying sources and funding strategies for varying types of SPHM technology.

## Standard 3. Incorporate Ergonomic Design Principles to Provide a Safe Environment of Care

The employer and healthcare workers partner to incorporate ergonomic design principles, such as the Prevention through Design (PtD) national initiative led by the National Institute for Occupational Safety and Health (NIOSH). Ergonomic design principles use a systematized and proactive process to prevent or reduce occupationally related illnesses, fatalities, and exposures by including prevention considerations in all designs that affect individuals in the occupational environment.

### 3.1 EMPLOYERS

**3.1.1 Plan for a safe environment of care during new construction and/or renovation**

Construction and/or remodeling will incorporate the review of ergonomic and other safety and health risk factors into the design of the project. This includes the design of facilities, process flow, evaluation of different technology, and accessibility issues.

**3.1.2 Include diverse perspectives related to ergonomic design principles**

Input will be gathered from healthcare workers and ancillary/support staff at all stages and in all activities of new construction, rebuilding, and remodeling.

> **IN DAILY PRACTICE ...**
>
> SUSAN, A 57-YEAR-OLD RN, WORKS at the old community hospital. "I am proud to work in an under-served community. We never have enough money, but we get by. I do worry about injury, for both me and my patients. The rooms are crowded and the bathrooms are small, with tight corners. We can't keep the portable lift in the hallway because of fire code, so it is kept in the far storeroom—it might as well be on the moon. We just don't use it. I hear that we are getting remodeled. I sure hope they fix things."
>
> *(See also Standards 1, 2, 4, and 8.)*

### 3.2 HEALTHCARE WORKER

**3.2.1 Provide input into the design**

The healthcare worker and ancillary/support staff will provide input into the design of construction and remodeling projects.

**CONSIDERATIONS FOR COMMUNITY SETTINGS**

Ergonomic design principles must be applied in any healthcare setting undergoing construction or renovation.

## Standard 4. Select, Install, and Maintain SPHM Technology

The employer and healthcare workers partner to incorporate appropriate SPHM technology for the program. Such a program provides the assistive tools within the organization and at point of care that are used to facilitate SPHM, thus minimizing the risk of injury to both the healthcare recipient and the healthcare worker. SPHM technology may include equipment, devices, accessories, software, and multimedia resources.

**4.1 EMPLOYER**

**4.1.1 Perform an organizational SPHM technology needs assessment**
An interprofessional group of stakeholders and/or subject-matter experts will perform the organization's SPHM technology needs assessment within all environments of care.

**4.1.2 Develop a plan for the selection of SPHM technology**
A plan will be identified to ensure that SPHM technology meets quality and safety standards and that devices and accessories are compatible and interoperable within the organization or facility.

**4.1.3 Provide opportunities for trial and provide feedback about SPHM technology**
The organization considering the purchase or rental of SPHM technology will provide healthcare workers with opportunities to try out the technology and provide feedback.

**4.1.4 Develop a SPHM technology procurement plan and introduction schedule**
The SPHM technology procurement plan and introduction schedule will be developed and communicated to the healthcare worker.

**4.1.5 Provide and strategically place SPHM technology for accessibility**
The organization will develop a process for providing SPHM technology that ensures ease in accessibility. The quantity and type of SPHM technology will be sufficient to minimize risk for the healthcare recipient population served and the environment of care.

> **IN DAILY PRACTICE ...**
>
> SALLY WANTS CEILING LIFTS AND ALGO-RITHMS for her facility. "I visited a Veterans Health Administration hospital and saw how they used ceiling lifts to reposition patients in bed and to safely ambulate them to the bathroom or a walk in the hall. Algorithms could help us consistently get our patients up early and often, and I'll bet that we could achieve our goal of zero falls and zero pressure ulcers. In fact, I'll bet that would help on several of our NDNQI measures."
>
> *(See also Standards 2, 6, and 8.)*

**4.1.6 Install fixed SPHM technology according to manufacturer's specifications**
Fixed SPHM technology, such as ceiling or wall-mounted lifts, or bariatric toilets, will be installed according to the manufacturer's specifications.

**4.1.7 Establish a system to clean, disinfect, maintain, repair, and upgrade SPHM technology**
The employer will develop procedures for regular cleaning, disinfection, and maintenance. SPHM technology will be maintained and repaired per manufacturer's specifications. The responsibility for monitoring, and acting on, upgrade or recall notices for equipment or software will be assigned to a specific position.

**4.2 HEALTHCARE WORKER**

**4.2.1 Participate in the SPHM technology needs assessment**
The healthcare worker will participate in the SPHM technology needs assessment and other processes, as appropriate.

**4.2.2 Participate in SPHM technology selection**
The healthcare worker will participate in the selection of technology as appropriate.

**CONSIDERATIONS FOR COMMUNITY SETTINGS**
A subject-matter expert in SPHM technology can provide solutions for specific problems, or develop solutions for an entire organization. The SPHM technology industry continues to develop new technologies, work practices, and systems to meet the needs of users across the continuum of care. Newer technologies solve age-old problems like narrow doorways, small bathrooms, low beds, and steps. Healthcare recipients and their families must be encouraged to provide input regarding the usability, usefulness, and desirability of the SPHM technology options available to them.

## Standard 5. Establish a System for Education, Training, and Maintaining Competence

The employer and healthcare workers partner to establish an effective system of education and training to maintain SPHM competence of healthcare workers and ancillary/support staff.

### 5.1 EMPLOYER

**5.1.1 Establish an education and training system**

SPHM education and training will be provided to the healthcare worker and ancillary/support staff as appropriate, at orientation, annually, and with the introduction of new competencies or technology solutions. Select a methodology that meets the needs of the adult learner.

> **IN DAILY PRACTICE ...**
>
> SHERRIE ROLLED HER EYES. OFF THE floor again! She hoped that the SPHM training would go quickly, because they were short of staff anyway. Maybe if she signed in and stayed for just a few minutes. . . .
>
> *(See also Standards 1 and 2.)*

**5.1.2 Include healthcare workers from across the continuum of care**

The content of the education and training will be specific to the role and setting of the healthcare worker or ancillary/support staff.

**5.1.3 Provide time for employees to participate in learning sessions**

Employee participation will be facilitated by providing time and scheduling support services. Education and training will be provided during scheduled work hours, including shift work.

**5.1.4 Provide appropriate SPHM technology for education and training**

Interactive education and training will be conducted using the same types of SPHM technology used for healthcare recipient care within the organization. Simulation or point-of-care training is preferred.

**5.1.5 Require and document healthcare worker competence**

The healthcare worker will demonstrate competence with SPHM prior to providing actual care. The effectiveness of the education and training will be monitored.

**5.1.6 Provide time and resources for education of healthcare recipients**

The organization will allocate time and learning resources for healthcare workers to educate healthcare recipients and their families about SPHM, as appropriate.

## 5.2 HEALTHCARE WORKER

### 5.2.1 Establish and maintain competence

The healthcare worker will actively participate in education and training to maintain competence related to SPHM, and serve as a role model for safe behavior.

### 5.2.2 Engage and educate the healthcare recipient regarding SPHM

The healthcare worker will engage and educate healthcare recipients, family, community, and co-workers in a manner that is easily understood by the learner.

### CONSIDERATIONS FOR COMMUNITY SETTINGS

Healthcare workers employed in community settings such as home health agencies, congregant care, or schools may encounter a wide variety of SPHM technology. When new SPHM technology will be used, training should be provided at the point of care, and the employer must ensure that the healthcare worker has access to a subject-matter expert for questions or consultation. Periodic orientations with SPHM technology vendors or a local durable medical goods vendor may be helpful and would provide a time for evaluative feedback on the special needs of community settings.

## Standard 6. Integrate Patient-Centered SPHM Assessment, Plan of Care, and Use of SPHM Technology

The employer and healthcare workers partner to adapt the plan of care to meet the SPHM needs of individual healthcare recipients and specify appropriate SPHM technology and methods.

### 6.1 EMPLOYER

**6.1.1 Provide a written procedure on the SPHM assessment and plan of care**

The written procedure outlines how to evaluate a healthcare recipient's SPHM status, establish goals, select technology for specific care tasks, and address roles and responsibilities of the healthcare worker related to assessment and scoring, evaluation, plan of care, and documentation.

**6.1.2 Require initial and ongoing assessment or process to determine SPHM needs**

The healthcare recipient will be evaluated for physical, cognitive, clinical, and rehabilitative needs that impact mobility needs, both initially and on an ongoing basis. The outcome of the assessment, evaluation, or scoring system will be incorporated within the individual plan of care.

**6.1.3 Include SPHM in the plan of care**

The individual plan of care will specify required SPHM technology and methods and expected outcomes. The plan of care should promote independence, as appropriate.

**6.1.4 Address SPHM at transitions of care**

The shift report, transfer, or discharge plan will include information and resources for SPHM, as appropriate.

**6.1.5 Provide a system to resolve healthcare recipient's refusal**

A system will be developed to address the safety of the healthcare worker and the healthcare recipient if the healthcare recipient refuses the use of SPHM technology.

---

**IN DAILY PRACTICE ...**

MILDRED AND BERT WERE HIGH SCHOOL sweethearts and have been married 50 years. Now they are facing a long recovery following Bert's stroke. "I just don't know what I am going to do. I want to take care of him at home, but I don't think I can get him out of bed or onto the toilet by myself. I really don't want to put him in a nursing home. He needs me, I need him, it will wipe out our savings, and we'll probably lose our home. I wish someone would talk to me."

*(See also Standards 1 and 5.)*

---

### 6.1.6 Monitor healthcare recipient injuries associated with patient handling and mobility

The organization will determine the frequency, severity, and cost of healthcare recipient injuries associated with patient handling and mobility.

### 6.1.7 Support safe delegation of SPHM tasks and activities

The organization will support the delegation or assignment in a manner consistent with its state's individual practice act or other legislation governing licensure.

## 6.2 HEALTHCARE WORKER

### 6.2.1 Perform initial and ongoing assessment of mobility and SPHM needs

The healthcare worker will perform initial and ongoing assessments of mobility and SPHM needs, as per organizational policy.

### 6.2.2 Communicate with the healthcare recipient and family

The healthcare worker will teach the healthcare recipient and family, as appropriate, about the purposes and safe use of SPHM technology.

### 6.2.3 Address SPHM at transitions of care

The healthcare worker will include SPHM in shift reports, transfer reports, and discharge planning.

### 6.2.4 Delegate care tasks in a safe manner

The healthcare worker will ensure that delegation or assignment of SPHM tasks is completed in a manner consistent with state professional practice acts or other applicable laws or regulations.

### CONSIDERATIONS FOR COMMUNITY SETTINGS

The healthcare worker will provide information on appropriate and available SPHM technologies and supplies. Healthcare recipients and their families must be central to the process of selection. Helping the family understand the importance of the SPHM technology is critical in obtaining their "buy-in." The use of SPHM technology in long-term care, and specifically in assisted living settings, is an important part of promoting independence. A progression through different technologies may indicate a functional change: possibly deterioration, possibly improvement.

## Standard 7. Include SPHM in Reasonable Accommodation and Post-Injury Return to Work

The employer and healthcare workers partner to establish a comprehensive SPHM program that can help the employer provide reasonable accommodations to healthcare workers who were injured.

### 7.1 EMPLOYER

#### 7.1.1 Facilitate the employment of disabled workers

The organization will have a system to match the physical capability of an injured healthcare worker to the physical demands of a job. The use of SPHM technology is one strategy to facilitate the employment of disabled or injured workers.

#### 7.1.2 Monitor healthcare worker injuries associated with patient handling and mobility

Monitoring will include determining the frequency, severity, and cost of healthcare worker injuries associated with lifting, transfers, repositioning, and mobility. Data about healthcare worker injuries will be used to prevent future injuries. The frequency, severity, and cost of patient handling and mobility injuries included in the worker's compensation program will be carefully monitored.

> **IN DAILY PRACTICE ...**
>
> LYDIA IS A PHYSICAL THERAPIST AT General Hospital. "I hate to see my co-workers injured while lifting, repositioning, or ambulating patients. The amazing thing is that a lot of the injuries happen when working with relatively small, frail patients. I guess the workers forget. Part of my job is getting them healthy enough for early return to work. People heal better if they are active and feel needed. I work with them on using the SPHM equipment correctly and consistently. Frankly, I wish it was used all the time."
>
> *(See also Standards 1, 2, 4, and 5.)*

#### 7.1.3 Facilitate early return to work following injury

The employer will establish, implement, and sustain a process to help injured healthcare workers return to work as quickly as possible to jobs that are medically suited to their needs. The process will be managed to ensure that restrictions are honored, preventing harm and expediting recovery during the restricted work activity period.

### 7.2 HEALTHCARE WORKER

#### 7.2.1 Notify the employer of physical limitations or restrictions

The healthcare worker will notify the employer of any physical limitations and provide up-to-date medical documentation of physical limitations or restrictions.

### 7.2.2 Participate in the return to work plan

The injured healthcare worker will be accountable for complying with the medical treatment plan and for returning to work in a role that accommodates medical restrictions.

### CONSIDERATIONS FOR COMMUNITY SETTINGS

Every healthcare organization will have a system for evaluating, managing, and reducing healthcare worker injuries.

## Standard 8. Establish a Comprehensive Evaluation System

The employer and healthcare workers partner to establish a comprehensive system to evaluate SPHM program status, using staff performance, staff injury incidence and severity, and healthcare recipient outcome metrics.

### 8.1 EMPLOYERS

#### 8.1.1 Establish a comprehensive evaluation system

The organization will establish a comprehensive evaluation and quality improvement system during the planning phase, based on the goals and objectives of the SPHM program. Formative and summative evaluations will be performed, including process and outcome measures. Evaluations will be conducted on a regular basis.

The program evaluation methods will change depending on the maturity of the SPHM program. A mechanism will be used to provide organizational leadership and key stakeholders with the results of these analyses. Positive outcomes will be emphasized and remediation plans will be developed for substandard outcomes.

#### 8.1.2 Identify a variety of data sources and measures

The organization will identify appropriate quality improvement indicators that reflect the content of *Safe Patient Handling and Mobility: Interprofessional National Standards,* assess the effectiveness of the SPHM program and the processes implemented during program development, and identify selected program outcomes.

#### 8.1.3 Utilize evidence-based methods for data collection and analysis

The organization will use standardized definitions and evidence-based methods for data collection and analysis. Evaluation methods may change depending on the maturity of the SPHM program.

#### 8.1.4 Disseminate findings

The organization establishes a formal process of informing all stakeholders of the SPHM outcomes using a variety of techniques, including, but not limited to, online summary of data; printed materials distributed to the healthcare worker; and regularly scheduled staff meetings, management meetings, and organizational meetings (see Standard 1.1.5).

> **IN DAILY PRACTICE ...**
>
> STACY, THE CHIEF FINANCIAL OFFICER, was amazed. The Safe Patient Handling and Mobility Committee had turned in a concise and complete business plan for upgrading and expanding the SPHM technology. "They used a new method for calculating the return on investment that demonstrated ranges of direct and indirect costs. They considered impact on worker's compensation, staff turnover, improved patient safety, and HCAP scores. They even gathered data on 30-day readmissions related to immobility and falls, and made recommendations for better discharge planning. With value-based purchasing, this is an investment I can support."
>
> *(See also Standards 2, 6, and 7.)*

### 8.1.5 Develop a plan for quality improvement and remediation of deficiencies

A diverse group of stakeholders (Standard 2.1.1) will review the data and develop recommendations. The organization will develop and implement a plan or activities to remediate deficiencies within a reasonable time.

### 8.1.6 Comply with the organization's policies, professional codes of ethics, privacy laws and regulations, and other regulatory language

The SPHM program will comply with organizational policies, appropriate professional codes of ethics, the Health Insurance Portability Privacy and Accountability Act, the Americans with Disabilities Act, state worker's compensation laws, and other applicable codes and regulations.

### 8.2 HEALTHCARE WORKER

### 8.2.1 Assist with data collection

The healthcare worker will provide accurate information during data collection and communication of results.

### 8.2.2 Comply with the organization's policies, professional codes of ethics, privacy laws and regulations, and other regulatory language

The healthcare worker will be accountable for knowing and following the policies of the organization, following a professional code of ethics, and respecting the privacy of co-workers and healthcare recipients.

### CONSIDERATIONS FOR COMMUNITY SETTINGS

Every healthcare organization will have a system for evaluating and improving the effectiveness of the SPHM program.

# Glossary

**ancillary/support staff.** Individuals whose work provides necessary support to the SPHM program. This may include consultants and staff members from departments such as risk management, safety, infection prevention, occupational health, transportation, security, activity direction, recreational therapy, creative art therapy, environmental services, laundry, volunteers, engineering, biomedical engineering, facilities, morgue, funeral home, purchasing, and contracting.

**assessment for SPHM.** Use of a scoring or other system to examine and evaluate the physical, mental, cognitive, medical, and/or environmental conditions of a healthcare recipient to determine appropriate SPHM methods, technology, and supplies. Assessment for SPHM may be an interprofessional activity, with collaboration from several disciplines.

**care plan.** See *plan of care.*

**community settings.** Nonhospital settings where healthcare interventions are performed, including, but not limited to, the healthcare recipient's home, long-term care, rehabilitation centers, assisted living, group homes, healthcare clinics, outpatient facilities, schools, prisons, and congregant and day care.

**competence.** An expected, measurable, and confirmed level of performance that integrates knowledge, skills, abilities, and judgment, based on established scientific knowledge and expectation for practice.

**continuum of care.** Health care received by the healthcare recipient on a continuing basis that is provided from the first point of contact through all phases of care.

**culture of safety.** Core values and behaviors resulting from a collective and sustained commitment by organizational leadership, managers, and healthcare workers to emphasize safety over competing goals.

**delegation.** The transfer of responsibility for the performance of a task from one individual to another, while retaining accountability for the outcome. The decision of whether or not to delegate is based upon professional judgment concerning the condition of the healthcare recipient, the competence of the individual being delegated to, and the degree of supervision that will be required.

**education.** The transfer of information to others in order to raise awareness and increase understanding of the subject. Includes relaying of information during orientation and in-service education.

**employer.** The healthcare organization, agency, system, corporation, business, or person(s) that employ or contract with the healthcare worker, at all levels of the continuum of care. The term *organization* is used interchangeably in these standards.

**environment of care.** Any environment in which care is being provided, such as prehospital care, hospital units, bariatrics, surgery, dental, rehabilitation, long-term care, assisted living, home care, hospice, ambulatory care, occupational health, group homes, schools, correctional facilities, morgues, and other settings.

**ergonomic design principles.** A systematized, proactive approach to prevent or reduce occupationally related illnesses, fatalities, and exposures by including prevention considerations in all construction and remodeling designs that impact individuals in the occupational environment.

**ergonomics.** The scientific discipline concerned with the understanding of interactions among humans and other elements of a work system. Such a system would include care tasks performed for the healthcare recipient, the physical and organizational environment where work is performed, and the tools used to help perform the work. Ergonomics encompasses the knowledge of human physical and cognitive abilities and limitations as applied to the design of work systems, organizations, job tasks, equipment, building components, and environments to prevent or reduce the risk of error and musculoskeletal and other injuries/disorders.

**essential physical functions.** The physical duties that a healthcare worker must be able to perform for a specific job, with or without reasonable accommodation.

**evaluation.** A comprehensive system to assess or analyze SPHM program status, using staff performance, healthcare recipient outcome metrics, and a mechanism to provide organizational leadership and key stakeholders with results from these analyses.

**formative evaluation.** A method of assessing the worth of a program while the program activities are in progress. A formative evaluation focuses on process.

**handling.** The use of the hands and/or assistive devices to perform an activity. Handling may involve either dynamic (movement) activities, such as repositioning, lifting/lowering, pushing/pulling, carrying, or turning; or static (stationary) activities, such as holding or supporting.

**healthcare recipient.** An individual who is receiving health care. In the context of these standards, they are individuals who are receiving health care that involves assistance with handling and mobility. This definition is inclusive of patients, clients, residents, students, individuals living in community settings, and others as appropriate. Patient families and volunteer caregivers are included.

**healthcare worker.** An individual involved in the provision of care to another individual and who works for the employer at any level in the continuum of care. Examples of healthcare workers include, but are not limited to, nurses, nursing assistants, resident assistants, home health aides, direct care workers working in community settings, occupational therapists, physical therapists, therapist assistants, radiology technologists, infection control practitioners, peer leaders, social workers, morgue personnel, emergency medical technicians, paramedics, and transporters, physicians, dentists, school teachers, and para-educators. Settings with organized labor should include union representation.

**high-risk tasks.** For the purposes of these standards, patient handling and mobility tasks characterized by biomechanical and postural stressors imposed on the healthcare worker.

**home care.** Services provided to individuals and families in their homes or residences. The care may be either supportive or custodial in nature, such as assistance with bathing, dressing, or feeding; or skilled care that requires the interventions of a licensed healthcare professional such as a nurse, therapist, or physician. Home care is unique among healthcare settings in that the healthcare worker is a guest in the healthcare recipient's home; therefore, the healthcare recipient and family have much greater control over how the plan of treatment is delivered.

**injury.** For the purposes of these standards, damage or harm to the healthcare worker or healthcare recipient as a result of patient handling and mobilization.

**interprofessional.** Reliant on the overlapping knowledge, skills, and abilities of each professional team member. Interprofessionalism can drive synergistic effects by which outcomes are enhanced and become more comprehensive than a simple aggregation of the individual efforts of the team members.

**long-term care.** Medical and nonmedical services provided to people with a chronic illness or disability who cannot care for themselves for long periods of time. Long-term care can be provided at home, in the community, in assisted living facilities, or in nursing homes.

**manager/management.** Defined for the purpose of these standards as middle and frontline management, such as nurse managers, radiology supervisors, and operational leaders (among others), who ensure application of policies and procedures.

**mobility.** Defined for the purpose of these standards as the progressive and active maintenance of, or increase in, physical activity of a healthcare recipient with or without assistance of healthcare worker action and SPHM technology.

**musculoskeletal disorder (MSD).** An injury or disorder of the muscles, nerves, tendons, joints, or cartilage, and disorder of the nerves, tendons, muscles, and supporting structures of the upper and lower limbs, neck, and lower back that are caused, precipitated, or exacerbated by sudden exertion or prolonged exposure to physical factors such as repetition, force, vibration, or awkward posture. This definition specifically excludes conditions such as fractures, contusions, abrasions, and lacerations resulting from sudden physical contact of the body with external objects (NIOSH, 2012).

**nonpunitive environment.** An environment that fosters trust to encourage healthcare workers to disclose healthcare errors so that the precursors to errors can be better understood and remedied. Healthcare workers know that they are accountable for their actions, but will not be held accountable for problems within the system or environment that are beyond their control.

**organization.** The healthcare organization, agency, system, corporation, business, or person(s) that employ or contract with the healthcare worker at all levels of the continuum of care. The term *employer* is used interchangeably in these standards.

**organizational leadership.** Defined for the purpose of these standards as the high-level, senior leaders of the employer, such as the chief officer(s), president, vice president(s), or others with significant strategic or operational roles.

**patient.** See *healthcare recipient*.

**patient handling injury.** A healthcare worker injury due to healthcare recipient handling and mobility activities.

**peer leader.** A staff member who receives special education and training on SPHM and use of technology. Peer leaders are the SPHM subject-matter expert in their clinical units/areas and share knowledge and skills with co-workers, management, and healthcare recipients. Peer leaders foster knowledge transfer and forge a direct connection between staff and program goals. This term is commonly used in Veterans Administration care settings.

**plan of care.** An individualized, written, patient-centered handling and mobilization plan based on an assessment or use of a scoring system of the healthcare recipient's capabilities, needs, and goals. The SPHM plan of care is incorporated into the overall plan of care.

**return to work program.** A program designed and administered to safely return individuals who have sustained injuries or illnesses to the work environment, in a full or transitional capacity, as quickly as is medically advisable. The goal of the program is to enhance worker recovery and/or rehabilitation, minimize direct and indirect costs associated with work injury or illness, and prevent service interruption.

**right of refusal.** The right of the healthcare worker to refuse an assignment, or a healthcare recipient to refuse a treatment or the use of SPHM technology. See Appendix A (Standards 1.1.3 and 6.1.5) for more information.

**safe patient handling and mobility (SPHM) program.** A formal, systematized program for reducing the risk of injuries and MSDs for healthcare workers, fostering a culture of safety while improving the quality of care and reducing the risk of physical injury to healthcare recipients.

**simulation.** Imitation of the operation of a system. For example, SPHM techniques may be simulated by using technology to lift a mannequin or another healthcare worker instead of lifting a healthcare recipient.

**subject-matter expert.** A person who exhibits the highest level of expertise in performing a specialized job, task, or skill set. Examples include those with advanced knowledge of ergonomics, industrial hygiene, human factors, and biomechanics.

**summative evaluation.** A method of assessing the worth of a program at the end of the program activities. A summative evaluation focuses on outcomes.

**technology.** The assistive tools used, within the organization and at the point of care, to facilitate the healthcare worker's performance of SPHM tasks, thus minimizing the risk of injury to the healthcare recipient and the healthcare worker. Technology may include equipment, devices, accessories, software, and multimedia resources.

**technology needs assessment.** An assessment done by using ergonomic principles of evaluation. The assessment includes evaluation of the physical, mental, and cognitive characteristics of the healthcare recipient or population, and the physical environment of care in which care is being delivered, so as to recommend appropriate SPHM methods and technology.

**training.** The process of bringing a person to an agreed standard of proficiency by hands-on practice or simulation applications.

# Appendix A. Evaluative Tools, Strategies, and Resources

Successful implementation of SPHM programs requires the commitment of both employers and healthcare workers. However, the evaluation measures listed here align with the standards specific to the employer because it is the employer that is responsible for overseeing the development, implementation, evaluation, remediation, and maintenance of SPHM programs.

The purpose of this appendix is to begin to identify tools, strategies, and resources to support implementation and evaluation of the standards. The following list is not comprehensive, nor is it intended to be prescriptive.

## STANDARD 1. ESTABLISH A CULTURE OF SAFETY

| Standard | Evaluation questions | Tools, strategies, resources |
|---|---|---|
| *1.1.1 Establish a statement of commitment to a culture of safety.*<br><br>Organizational policy will include a written commitment to a culture of safety that will be used to guide the organization's priorities, resource allocation, policies, and procedures. The written statement regarding SPHM will describe layers of accountability across sectors and settings. | Do the organization and healthcare workers promote a culture of safety? | The culture of safety must be evaluated within units or work areas, and the organization as a whole, to identify psychosocial factors, such as relationship dynamics within the department, staffing shortages, and staff and management attitudes toward healthcare worker and healthcare recipient safety. The goal is to identify the readiness for culture change (that is, a change in practice related to lifting and moving of healthcare recipients) and potential barriers that must be addressed in order to successfully implement an effective SPHM program.<br>　A validated survey tool should be used to assess the culture of safety. The Johns Hopkins Center for Innovation in Quality Patient Care maintains a web site on safety culture in health care with strategies for measurement.<br><br>　Developing a culture of safety requires the implementation of a comprehensive health and safety management system, and SPHM would be one component of that system. Examples of occupational health and safety management systems resources include:<br>　ANSI/AIHA Z10-2012, *Occupational Safety and Health Management Systems*<br>　BSI-OHSAS 18001, *Occupational Health and Safety Management Systems*<br>　National Safety Council, *Safety and Health Code of Ethics Resource Guide: How to Implement a Code of Ethics for Safety and Health in Your Organization*<br>　OSHA Voluntary Protection Program |

| Standard | Evaluation questions | Tools, strategies, resources |
| --- | --- | --- |
| *1.1.2 Establish a nonpunitive environment.*<br><br>Organizational policy will support a system to encourage healthcare workers to report hazards, errors, incidents, and accidents, so that the precursors to SPHM errors can be better understood and organizational issues can be changed to prevent future incidents and injuries. Healthcare workers know that they are accountable for their actions, but will not be held accountable for problems within the system or environment that are beyond their control. | Are healthcare workers able to report hazards or errors without fear of retribution?<br><br>When healthcare workers are held accountable, does the organization consider how deficiencies in organizational systems contributed to the error?<br><br>When healthcare workers report hazards or errors, does the organization analyze the issue to identify and then correct hazards associated with patient handling and mobility? | The ANA position statement "Just Culture" provides guidance for the application of Just Culture for nursing and health care in a variety of settings (ANA, 2010).<br><br>A scholarly paper on validated tools for Just Culture in the healthcare environment can be found on the NCBI web site (Frankel, Leonard, & Denham, 2006). |
| *1.1.3 Provide a system for right of refusal.*<br><br>Organizational policy will provide the healthcare worker the right to accept, reject, or object to any healthcare recipient transfer, repositioning, or mobility assignment that puts the healthcare recipient or the healthcare worker at risk for injury. The refusal shall be made in writing, without fear of retribution. The policy will describe steps for resolving the hazard. | Does the organization have a policy and procedure for healthcare workers to report an unsafe assignment, and refuse the unsafe assignment prior to assuming responsibility? | The ANA position statement "Patient Safety: Rights of Registered Nurses When Considering a Patient Assignment" lists recommendations for nurses, the employer/healthcare agency, the patient, and the consumer (ANA, 2009). |

| Standard | Evaluation questions | Tools, strategies, resources |
|---|---|---|
| *1.1.4 Provide safe levels of staffing.*<br><br>An evidence-based system will be used to determine safe and appropriate caseloads. Adequate staffing levels will support safe patient handling and mobility, including allocated time for training and education. | Does the organization use a system for safe staffing? | The publication *ANA's Principles of Nurse Staffing* provides guidance (ANA, 2012b). |
| *1.1.5 Establish a system for communication and collaboration.*<br><br>Collaboration among all sectors and settings is critical. The organization will utilize a variety of communication systems to inform and engage the healthcare workers and healthcare recipients about SPHM. | Does the organization have communication systems to inform and engage healthcare workers about SPHM?<br><br>Is collaboration among sectors and settings evident?<br><br>Are there effective communication strategies to facilitate the ongoing engagement of healthcare workers within specific settings? | Organizational communications must address each of the eight standards. Principles of adult learning will be considered when developing communications. Healthcare workers must be able to describe how to submit ideas; report hazards, incidents, accidents, and near misses; and who to ask if there are questions about the SPHM program.<br><br>Collaborative and collegial efforts between sectors and settings, such as committees or task forces, must include the perspectives of organizational leadership, healthcare workers, ancillary/support staff, and healthcare recipients, as appropriate. Organizational units or specific settings may need their own internal communication systems about SPHM, such as management reports or safety huddles. Positive communication, such as celebrating quick wins or small successes, is an important strategy to build the support of healthcare workers.<br><br>The Joint Commission report on improving patient and worker safety contains a section (2.5.3) on tools for improving safety communication (TJC, 2012). |

## STANDARD 2. IMPLEMENT AND SUSTAIN A SAFE PATIENT HANDLING AND MOBILITY (SPHM) PROGRAM

| Standard | Evaluation | Tools, strategies, resources |
|---|---|---|
| *2.1.1 Designate a group or groups of stakeholders to develop, implement, evaluate, remediate, and maintain a SPHM program.*<br><br>An organizational committee will identify or develop systems that support SPHM programs. The committee will receive and review data about SPHM and make recommendations for improvement. The work of the committee will reflect collaboration among organizational leadership, the healthcare worker, and ancillary/support workers. | Is the committee responsible for SPHM composed of a diverse group of stakeholders? | Committees, task forces, and other groups will be evaluated for interprofessional and interdepartmental involvement, as appropriate to the purposes of the organization. A core group of stakeholders will be assigned to work on the issues over a period of time, and involve others on an as-needed basis.<br><br>Examples of participants include organizational leadership, management, healthcare workers, ancillary/support staff, healthcare recipients, families, and volunteer caregivers, as appropriate.<br><br>The Veterans Health Administration peer leader program is one example of a stakeholder structure that supports SPHM. A plan is established to replace core SPHM committee members and/or peer leaders so as to ensure sustainability and continuity of the SPHM program (VISN 8, 2013). |
| *2.1.2 Perform a comprehensive assessment of SPHM.*<br><br>The organization will initially and periodically perform a comprehensive assessment of patient handling, mobility, and technology, including a SPHM technology needs assessment (see Standard 4.1.1). | Was there an initial, comprehensive, written needs/ergonomic assessment to define the scope and direction of the SPHM program?<br><br>Are periodic needs assessments accomplished? | Evaluation of the elements and effectiveness of SPHM can be done using the data sources matched to each standard in this appendix. Nelson et al. described the development and evaluation of a multifaceted ergonomics program to prevent injuries associated with patient handling and mobility tasks (Nelson, A. M., et al., 2008). The PHAMA white paper also contains criteria for SPHM assessment (FGI, 2010b).<br><br>A purpose of the assessment is to proactively identify and address risk factors that may be present that increase the risk for healthcare recipient or healthcare worker injury. |

| Standard | Evaluation | Tools, strategies, resources |
|---|---|---|
| *2.1.3 Develop a written SPHM program, with goals, objectives, and a plan for ongoing evaluation, compliance, and quality improvement.*<br><br>The written SPHM program will address each of the Safe Patient Handling and Mobility Interprofessional National Standards, and will reflect compliance with federal, state, and local laws and regulations. The written program will include short- and long-term goals and objectives, and a realistic plan and timeline to meet the goals and evaluation requirements. The written SPHM program will identify, by title, those individuals who have responsibility, authority, and accountability for developing and implementing the plan. The written SPHM program also will establish a clear reporting hierarchy to monitor compliance. | Are there specific and measurable goals for the reduction or elimination of healthcare worker and healthcare recipient injury, and the data sources to track the progress toward those goals?<br><br>Is a management tool in place to evaluate program compliance and status as related to the written plan? | The written plan will include short- and long-term goals and objectives for the SPHM program. The goals will be prioritized and incorporated into a realistic plan and timeline. |
| *2.1.4 Customize and integrate the SPHM program across the continuum of care.*<br><br>The SPHM program will be customized for, and integrated into, care settings throughout the organization and continuum of care, ensuring that SPHM is addressed through transitions of care. | Are the SPHM needs of specific settings identified?<br>Is each setting-specific plan appropriately integrated into the organizational SPHM program? | Establish a plan for each setting with patient handling and mobility hazards, and a baseline from which to evaluate the effectiveness of the SPHM program. Goals for the specific setting will relate to the organizational goals (see Standard 2.1.3). |

| Standard | Evaluation | Tools, strategies, resources |
|---|---|---|
| *2.1.5 Provide funding to implement and sustain the program.*<br><br>The employer will identify and allocate funding to implement and sustain the program based on business-case and return-on-investment analytics or cost/benefit analysis. | Does the budget specify funding for the SPHM program?<br><br>Was a cost/benefit analysis done? | Evaluate the capital and operating budgets for inclusion of each element of the organizational SPHM plan. This will include, but is not limited to, the cost to establish the program, the procurement of appropriate amounts/types of SPHM technology, maintenance, training, education, and updating as needed.<br><br>The organization may perform a cost/benefit analysis. The Facilities Guidelines Institute provides an overview of tools to determine ROI (FGI, 2010a). |
| *2.1.6 Identify the essential physical functions and high-risk tasks of jobs.*<br><br>The organization will identify the essential physical functions of a job in a written job description. An evidenced-based process or review of scientific literature will be used to identify activities that place the healthcare worker at high risk for injury. | Is there a systematic approach for identifying essential functions of healthcare worker jobs?<br><br>Have these essential functions related to patient handling and mobility been evaluated to determine if they are high risk, or has a review of scientific literature been conducted to gather information specific to each environment of care? | Strategies for identifying the tasks that put healthcare workers at high risk include use of ergonomic assessment and evaluation tools, literature reviews, analysis of incident and accident reports, and interviews with healthcare workers and organizational leadership.<br>    Ergonomic or other needs assessments used to determine high-risk tasks are performed initially; when occupational injuries or incidents related to patient handling and mobility tasks are reported; when a job, task, or process substantially changes; when healthcare recipient population characteristics change; when new jobs are introduced; at concept stage related to introduction of new SPHM technology or clinical or work processes; and when redesign of existing or building of new workspaces and facilities takes place.<br><br>*Ergonomics: Manual Handling of People in the Healthcare Sector* contains evaluations that can be used by trained professionals to determine the risk of functions of jobs (ISO, 2012). Several postural analysis and biomechanical tools have been used to assess physical stress in healthcare tasks.<br><br>(cont'd on pg. 52) |

| Standard | Evaluation | Tools, strategies, resources |
|---|---|---|
| | | (cont'd from pg. 53)<br><br>Some are used to diagnose problems as well as evaluate changes (Hignett, Fray, & Matz, 2012).<br><br>The Rapid Entire Body Assessment is a quick guide for evaluating injury risk (REBA, 2012).<br><br>An evaluation of a best-practices musculoskeletal injury prevention program in nursing homes is included in an article published in *Injury Prevention* (Collins, Wolf, Bell, & Evanoff, 2004).<br><br>The PHAMA includes a description of a patient care ergonomic evaluation (FGI, 2010b). |
| *2.1.7 Reduce the physical requirements of high-risk tasks.*<br><br>The organization will focus on reducing the physical requirements of high-risk healthcare recipient transfer, repositioning, and mobilization, and other applicable tasks through engineering, safe work practice, and/or administrative controls. | Can the organization demonstrate modification of high-risk SPHM tasks through engineering, safe work practices, and/or administrative controls? | Consider the task of repositioning a healthcare recipient in bed. An example of an administrative control is to replace the lift sheets (historically used for manual repositioning) with engineering controls such as appropriate SPHM technology and/or supplies.<br><br>A safe work practice would be to provide training and promote the use of available SPHM technology. |

## STANDARD 3. INCORPORATE ERGONOMIC DESIGN PRINCIPLES
## TO PROVIDE A SAFE ENVIRONMENT OF CARE

| Standard | Evaluation topics | Tools, strategies, resources |
|---|---|---|
| *3.1.1 Plan for a safe environment of care during new construction and/or renovation.*<br><br>Construction and/or remodeling will incorporate the review of ergonomic and other safety and health risk factors into the design of the project. This includes the design of facilities, process flow, evaluation of different technology, and accessibility issues. | Does the organization require inclusion of ergonomic design principles in all construction and remodeling projects of healthcare recipient care areas? | The organization will have a procedure to include ergonomic design principles in all construction and remodeling projects in healthcare recipient care areas. Examples of ergonomic design principles include:<br><br>■ Ensuring proper reinforcement of the floor and ceiling when installing ceiling lifts<br><br>■ Accessible storage of SPHM technology to keep hallways cleared for evacuation purposes.<br><br>■ Accessible storage of slings and other supplies on shelves between knee and shoulder height.<br><br>■ Accessible showers or tubs to facilitate bathing.<br><br>■ Wider doorways.<br><br>■ Bathrooms large enough to facilitate the use of wheelchairs or SPHM technology and fewer corners to negotiate when entering the bathroom.<br><br>■ Floor coverings that are easy to clean and not slippery when wet.<br><br>Information related to incorporating ergonomic design principles can be found in NIOSH's *Prevention through Design: Plan for the National Initiative* (NIOSH, 2010) and the *American National Standard: Prevention through Design—Guidelines for Addressing Occupational Hazards and Risks in Design and Redesign Processes* (ANSI/ASSE, 2011). |

| Standard | Evaluation topics | Tools, strategies, resources |
|---|---|---|
| *3.1.2 Include diverse perspectives related to ergonomic design principles.*<br><br>Input will be gathered from healthcare workers and ancillary/support staff at all stages and in all activities of new construction, rebuilding, and remodeling. | Are frontline healthcare recipients and ancillary/support staff included in planning for construction and remodeling? | Healthcare workers will be asked about challenges in their current environment and any ideas they have for improving safety and efficiency. A walk-through with the architect can help inform the project. |

## STANDARD 4. SELECT, INSTALL, AND MAINTAIN SPHM TECHNOLOGY

| Standard | Evaluation topics | Tools, strategies, resources |
|---|---|---|
| 4.1.1 Perform an organizational SPHM technology needs assessment.<br><br>An interprofessional group of stakeholders and/or subject-matter experts will perform the organization's SPHM technology needs assessment within all environments of care. | Did the initial SPHM assessment determine the differing needs of unique environments of care and the types and quantities of SPHM technology needed? | The assessment will include the physical environment, patient characteristics, existing SPHM technology or systems, healthcare worker feedback, and results from the cost/benefit analysis. The assessment must determine the differing needs of specific care settings or patient care units. The special needs of bariatric patients must be included. A series of helpful tools for a SPHM technology needs or ergonomic assessment can be found in the PHAMA white paper (FGI, 2010b).<br><br>Evidence-based assessments, algorithms, or SPHM subject-matter expert can help determine the types and quantities of SPHM technologies needed. |
| 4.1.2 Develop a plan for the selection of SPHM technology.<br><br>A plan will be identified to ensure that SPHM technology meets quality and safety standards and that devices and accessories are compatible and interoperable within the organization or facility. | Is there a procedure to guide the procurement of SPHM technology? | The U.S. Department of Veterans Affairs' Safe Patient Handling and Movement Resource Page includes a technology resource guide (VISN 8, 2013).<br><br>Appendix G of FGI's PHAMA white paper includes detailed guidance regarding the evaluation and selection of equipment (FGI, 2010b). |
| 4.1.3 Provide opportunities for trial and provide feedback about SPHM technology.<br><br>The organization considering the purchase or rental of SPHM technology will provide healthcare workers with opportunities to try out the technology and provide feedback. | Are healthcare workers able to provide feedback on SPHM technology being considered for procurement? | Technology fairs, and on-site pilot testing and evaluations, are strategies for engaging healthcare workers. Chapter 4 of the VA/DoD *Patient Care Ergonomic Resource Guide* includes product feature rating surveys for patient and staff evaluation of technology (VHA, 2013). |

| Standard | Evaluation topics | Tools, strategies, resources |
|---|---|---|
| *4.1.4 Develop a SPHM technology procurement plan and introduction schedule.*<br><br>The SPHM technology procurement plan and introduction schedule will be developed and communicated to the healthcare worker. | Is there a procurement plan and an introduction schedule for new SPHM technology? | The procurement plan will be based on the SPHM technology needs assessment and prioritized based on risk to healthcare workers and healthcare recipients. The procurement plan and introduction schedule must be communicated to healthcare workers. |
| *4.1.5 Provide and strategically place SPHM technology for accessibility.*<br><br>The organization will develop a process for providing SPHM technology and accessories that ensures ease in accessibility. The quantity and type of SPHM technology will be sufficient to minimize risk for the healthcare recipient population served and the environment of care. | Is the SPHM technology strategically placed for accessibility? | An evidence-based system will be used to determine the types and quantity of SPHM technology.<br><br>NIOSH established that in the nursing home setting, one full-body lift should be provided for every eight to ten non-weight-bearing residents and one stand-up lift should be provided for every eight to ten partially weight-bearing residents (NIOSH, 2010a).<br>    Hospitals are moving toward ceiling lifts in units where healthcare recipients are non-weight-bearing or partially weight-bearing.<br>    A professional with expertise related to SPHM technology will be consulted.<br><br>The placement and storage of SPHM technology will make the equipment accessible to the healthcare worker at the point of care, while maintaining compliance with Life Safety Code 101 (NFPA, 2000). |
| *4.1.6 Install fixed SPHM technology according to manufacturer's specifications.*<br><br>Fixed SPHM technology, such as ceiling- or wall-mounted lifts and bariatric toilets, will be installed according to the manufacturer's specifications. | Are there systems in place to ensure that ceiling lifts and other fixed SPHM technology are installed safely and according to manufacturer's specifications? | Compliance with manufacturer's specifications includes ensuring the architectural integrity of existing facilities to support the load of fixed SPHM technology. Any remodeling or construction will be done in accordance with Standard 3. |

| Standard | Evaluation topics | Tools, strategies, resources |
|---|---|---|
| *4.1.7 Establish a system to clean, disinfect, maintain, repair, and upgrade SPHM technology.* The employer will develop procedures for regular cleaning, disinfection, and maintenance. SPHM technology will be maintained and repaired per manufacturer's specifications. The responsibility for monitoring, and acting on, upgrade or recall notices for equipment or software will be assigned to a specific position. | Do support service systems effectively support the SPHM program? Are there systems for cleaning, disinfection, preventive maintenance, repair, and upgrades? Is there a system for monitoring recall notices? | Evaluate the capability of support service systems. such as environmental services, laundry services, facilities maintenance, and biomedical engineering, to support the SPHM program. Cleaning, disinfection, storage, and accessibility of slings may present operational challenges that will be worked out in advance of introduction and use. The SPHM technology vendor can help establish procedures for cleaning and disinfection of technology and supplies. Refer to the Centers for Disease Control and Prevention for more information about laundry and prevention of infection (CDC, 2011). The SPHM technology vendor will also assist with the recall of technology, supplies, and/or software. Refer to the U.S. Food and Drug Administration web site for more information about recalls (FDA, 2013). |

## STANDARD 5. ESTABLISH A SYSTEM FOR EDUCATION, TRAINING, AND MAINTAINING COMPETENCE

| Standard | Evaluation topics | Tools, strategies, resources |
|---|---|---|
| *5.1.1 Establish an education and training system.*<br><br>SPHM education and training will be provided to the healthcare worker and ancillary/support staff as appropriate, at orientation, annually, and with the introduction of new competencies or SPHM technology solutions. Select a methodology that meets the needs of the adult learner. | Is there a comprehensive assessment of the education and training of healthcare workers about SPHM?<br><br>Are competency assessments related to SPHM technology use required on a regular/annual basis? | Assessment of training will occur on a regular basis and will include assessment of healthcare worker proficiency in the use of all associated SPHM technology and methods. Consideration of the following is suggested: additional training needs, training structure/design, scheduling process, mechanism for staff feedback, and an effective system that tracks trained staff and competence achievement. Educators and trainers, managers, peer leaders, coaches, and others will use the principles of adult learning when instructing healthcare workers on SPHM.<br><br>O'Donnell developed an innovative teaching method that takes knowledge, attitude, and patient transfer skills from the simulation lab to the clinical setting (O'Donnell, J. G.-S., 2011) and an ergonomic protocol for patient transfer that can be taught using simulation methods (O'Donnell, J. G.-S., 2011).<br><br>The content can be reinforced in safety huddles, staff meetings, continuing education programs, and other formal or informal meetings.<br>    Healthcare workers who speak English as a second language will receive instruction using a method or language that facilitates learning.<br><br>Healthcare workers with increasing levels of responsibility may need additional education and/or training on general SPHM technology use, assessment, scoring tools, decision-making systems or algorithms, and the use of technology to promote progressive mobility and independent functioning. |

| Standard | Evaluation topics | Tools, strategies, resources |
|---|---|---|
| *5.1.2 Include healthcare workers from across the continuum of care.*<br><br>The content of the education and training should be specific to the role and setting of the healthcare worker or ancillary/support staff. | Are the education and training specific to the differing needs of all healthcare workers who perform patient handling and mobility tasks and the ancillary/support staff who support the program? | Education and training must be specific to the differing needs of various healthcare workers. |
| *5.1.3 Provide time for employees to participate in learning sessions.*<br><br>Employee participation will be facilitated by providing time and scheduling support services. Education and training should be provided during regular work hours, including shift work. | Are education and training provided during all shifts? Are healthcare workers allowed to attend? | Evaluate the ability of the healthcare worker to attend SPHM education and training during work hours. The healthcare worker will be paid for after-hours SPHM education and training.<br><br>Standard 1.1.4 addresses safe staffing; organizational leaders and managers may need to budget for additional healthcare worker hours to meet the needs of healthcare recipients during education and training sessions. |
| *5.1.4 Provide appropriate SPHM technology for education and training.*<br><br>Interactive education and training will be conducted using the same types of SPHM technology used for healthcare recipient care within the organization. Simulation or point-of-care training is preferred. | Is SPHM technology available for use during education and training? | Healthcare workers will be educated and trained using the same type of SPHM technology that will be used for healthcare recipient care. The training location will provide adequate room and not distract from ongoing healthcare recipient care. |
| *5.1.5 Require and document healthcare worker competence.*<br><br>The healthcare worker will demonstrate competence with SPHM prior to providing actual care. The effectiveness of the education and training will be monitored. | Is there a system to document the competence of healthcare workers on the understanding and use of technologies and methods for transfer, repositioning, ambulation, and other patient care tasks? | There must be a system to document the competence of healthcare workers on the understanding and use of technologies and methods for transfer, repositioning, ambulation, and other patient care tasks. |

| Standard | Evaluation topics | Tools, strategies, resources |
|---|---|---|
| *5.1.6 Provide time and resources for education of healthcare recipients.* The organization will allocate time and learning resources for healthcare workers to educate healthcare recipients and their families about SPHM, as appropriate. | Is time allocated for healthcare workers to educate healthcare recipients and their families about SPHM (as appropriate)? Does the organization provide learning resources appropriate to the healthcare recipient population? | The SPHM technology manufacturer may provide sample healthcare recipient education materials. |

## STANDARD 6. INTEGRATE PATIENT-CENTERED SPHM ASSESSMENT, PLAN OF CARE, AND USE OF SPHM TECHNOLOGY

| Standard | Evaluation topics | Tools, strategies, resources |
|---|---|---|
| *6.1.1 Provide a written procedure on the SPHM assessment and plan of care.*<br><br>The written procedure outlines how to evaluate a healthcare recipient's SPHM status, establish goals, select SPHM technology for specific care tasks, and address roles and responsibilities of the healthcare worker related to assessment and scoring, evaluation, plan of care, and documentation. | Is there a written procedure describing how to individually assess, evaluate, or score a healthcare recipient related to SPHM, establish a healthcare recipient's SPHM goals, and select appropriate SPHM technology? | Policy and procedure define the roles and responsibilities for all related staff and provide a reference for review when questions arise. The procedure will provide guidance on how to assess, evaluate, or score the healthcare recipient's needs and SPHM goals, and how to select SPHM technology appropriate for each individual healthcare recipient. The policy and procedure will also address SPHM technology availability, storage, function, and maintenance. |
| *6.1.2 Require initial and ongoing assessment or process to determine SPHM needs.*<br><br>The healthcare recipient will be evaluated for physical, cognitive, clinical, and rehabilitative needs that impact mobility needs, both initially and on an ongoing basis. The outcome of the assessment, evaluation, or scoring system will be incorporated within the individual plan of care. | Are healthcare recipients evaluated on a regular schedule for physical, cognitive, clinical, and rehabilitative needs that impact mobility and use of SPHM technology? | The mobility and SPHM assessments, evaluations, or scoring systems will be specific to the organizational setting and context. |

| Standard | Evaluation topics | Tools, strategies, resources |
|---|---|---|
| 6.1.3 Include SPHM in the plan of care.<br><br>The individual plan of care will specify required SPHM technology and methods and expected outcomes. The plan of care should promote independence, as appropriate. | Does the individual plan of care specify the required/recommended SPHM technology and methods? | The individual plan of care will specify the SPHM procedures, the required/recommended SPHM technology, and the parameters for its use.<br>    The selection of SPHM technology will be based on individual characteristics of the healthcare recipient; the goals of the activity; the results of the assessment, evaluation, or scoring system; and the use of algorithms or other decision-making tools. The SPHM technology must be safe, comfortable, efficient, and appropriate for the task or activity to be accomplished. |
| 6.1.4 Address SPHM at transitions of care.<br><br>The shift report, transfer, or discharge plan will include information and resources for SPHM, as appropriate. | Do the shift report within an organization and discharge plans relay information on SPHM, as appropriate? | The shift reports and discharge planning information will address the SPHM plan of care, level of dependence, and technology needed. |
| 6.1.5 Provide a system to resolve healthcare recipient's refusal.<br><br>A system will be developed to address the safety of the healthcare worker and the healthcare recipient if the healthcare recipient refuses the use of SPHM technology. | Is there a procedure to address the safety of both the healthcare worker and the healthcare recipient if the healthcare recipient refuses the use of SPHM technology? | A procedure must be in place to address the safety of both the healthcare worker and the healthcare recipient if the healthcare recipient refuses the use of SPHM technology. |

| Standard | Evaluation topics | Tools, strategies, resources |
|---|---|---|
| *6.1.6 Monitor health-care recipient injuries associated with patient handling and mobility.*<br><br>The organization will determine the frequency, severity, and cost of healthcare recipient injuries associated with patient handling and mobility. | Is there a system to monitor healthcare recipient injuries and clinical outcomes associated with patient handling and mobility? | Injuries to prevent include: falls, falls with injury, assisted falls, pressure ulcers,and complications of immobility.<br><br>Patient satisfaction surveys can be used to evaluate patient acceptance of SPHM technology and of SPHM tasks and activities.<br><br>Positive outcomes include prevention of other complications of immobility by early mobility, and healthcare recipient satisfaction as indicated on surveys. |
| *6.1.7 Support safe delegation of SPHM tasks and activities.*<br><br>The organization will support the delegation or assignment in a manner consistent with its state's individual practice act or other legislation governing licensure. | Do policies and practices support safe delegation of SPHM tasks and activities? | Policies and practices must support safe delegation of SPHM tasks and activities. |

## STANDARD 7. INCLUDE SPHM IN REASONABLE ACCOMMODATION AND POST-INJURY RETURN TO WORK

| Standard | Evaluation topics | Tools, strategies, resources |
|---|---|---|
| *7.1.1 Facilitate the employment of disabled workers.* <br><br> The organization will have a system to match the physical capability of an injured healthcare worker to the physical demands of a job. The use of SPHM technology is one strategy to facilitate the employment of disabled or injured workers. | Is SPHM technology available as an accommodation for a healthcare worker with an injury, as appropriate? | SPHM technology must be available as an accommodation for a healthcare worker with an injury, as appropriate. |
| *7.1.2 Monitor healthcare worker injuries associated with patient handling and mobility.* <br><br> Monitoring will include determining the frequency, severity, and cost of healthcare worker injuries associated with lifting, transfers, repositioning, and mobility. Data about healthcare worker injuries will be used to prevent future injuries. The frequency, severity, and cost of patient handling and mobility injuries included in the worker's compensation program will be carefully monitored. | Is there a system to monitor the frequency, severity, and costs of healthcare worker injuries associated with patient handling and mobility? | OSHA provides an online packet of forms and instructions for employers in regulated entities to record occupational illness and injury. The OSHA 300 Log is a primary resource for evaluation of a SPHM program. Entities not regulated by OSHA may be subject to a state plan or other industry-specific regulation, and will use a standard, accepted format for recording occupational injury and illness (OSHA, 2004). <br><br> Consistency in definitions, measures, and collection techniques is critical for obtaining meaningful, actionable data. <br><br> The Bureau of Labor Statistics (BLS) provides industry-wide comparative data on occupational injuries. The data can be used for benchmarking, although the government definitions should be compared closely with the organizational definitions. |

| Standard | Evaluation topics | Tools, strategies, resources |
|---|---|---|
| *7.1.3 Facilitate early return to work following injury.* <br><br> The employer will establish, implement, and sustain a process to help injured health-care workers return to work as quickly as possible to jobs that are medically suited to their needs. The process will be managed to ensure that restrictions are honored, preventing harm and expediting recovery during the restricted work activity period. | Is there a system to facilitate early return to work following injury, while honoring medical restrictions? | The organization may find consultation with a subject-matter expert helpful. Insurance brokers and companies that provide worker's compensation and/or disability insurance may employ people with expertise in return to work programs. |

## STANDARD 8. ESTABLISH A COMPREHENSIVE EVALUATION SYSTEM

| Standard | Evaluation topics | Tools, strategies, resources |
|---|---|---|
| *8.1.1 Establish a comprehensive evaluation system.*<br><br>The organization will establish a comprehensive evaluation and quality improvement system during the planning phase, based on the goals and objectives of the SPHM program. Formative and summative evaluations will be performed, including process and outcome measures. Evaluations will be conducted on a regular basis.<br>    The program evaluation methods will change depending on the maturity of the SPHM program. A mechanism will be used to provide organizational leadership and key stakeholders with the results of these analyses. Positive outcomes will be emphasized and remediation plans will be developed for substandard outcomes. | Are regular formative and summative evaluations performed, based on the goals of the SPHM program? | The written evaluation will provide answers to questions outlined in this appendix, as appropriate to the goals of the organization. The actual evaluation will be developed during the planning phase (Standard 2.1.3), and adapted over time based on progress toward an environment of care free of healthcare recipient or healthcare worker injury. |
| *8.1.2 Identify a variety of data sources and measures.*<br><br>The organization will identify appropriate quality improvement indicators that reflect the content of *SPHM Interprofessional National Standards*, assess the effectiveness of the SPHM | Do the data sources provide information on all eight standards? | Data sources should provide evaluative information on all eight standards. The Facilities Guidelines Institute's 2010 *Guidelines for the Design and Construction of Health Facilities* provides examples (FGI, 2010a). |

| Standard | Evaluation topics | Tools, strategies, resources |
|---|---|---|
| program and the processes implemented during program development, and identify selected program outcomes. | | |
| *8.1.3 Utilize evidence-based methods for data collection and analysis.*<br><br>The organization will use standardized definitions and evidence-based methods for data collection and analysis. Evaluation methods may change depending on the maturity of the SPHM program. | Does the organization use standardized definitions and consistent, evidence-based methods for data collection? | Standardized definitions are critical to ensure consistency of measures related to employee injury (Standard 7), and must be consistent over time. The organization will consult with its insurance company to help standardize descriptions of incidents, accidents, and lost-time accidents, and to clarify which incidents and accidents will be measured as associated with the SPHM program. The written evaluation will include any evidence of deviation from use of standardized definitions. For example, if the incident, accident, and worker's compensation reports were not analyzed to identify events related to SPHM, this will be noted. |
| *8.1.4 Disseminate findings.*<br><br>The organization establishes a formal process of informing all stakeholders of the SPHM outcomes using a variety of techniques, including, but not limited to, online summary of data; printed materials distributed to the healthcare worker; and regularly scheduled staff meetings, management meetings, and organizational meetings (see Standard 1.1.5). | Are there formal processes for informing stakeholders of the SPHM program outcomes? | A formal process must be in place for informing stakeholders of the SPHM program outcomes. |

| Standard | Evaluation topics | Tools, strategies, resources |
|---|---|---|
| *8.1.5 Develop a plan for quality improvement and remediation of deficiencies.*<br><br>A diverse group of stakeholders (Standard 2.1.1) will review the data and develop recommendations. The organization will develop and implement a plan or activities to remediate deficiencies within a reasonable time. | Does the SPHM committee or SPHM program manager recommend a plan to organizational leadership for quality improvement and remediation of deficiencies? | The SPHM committee or SPHM program manager must recommend a plan to organizational leadership for quality improvement and remediation of deficiencies. |
| *8.1.6 Comply with the organization's policies, professional codes of ethics, privacy laws and regulations, and other regulatory language.*<br><br>The SPHM program will comply with organizational policies, appropriate professional codes of ethics, the Health Insurance Portability Privacy and Accountability Act, the Americans with Disabilities Act, state worker's compensation laws, and other applicable codes and regulations. | Are organizational policies and practices consistent with a code of ethics, the law, privacy requirements, and other policies? | Organizational policies and practices must be consistent with a code of ethics, the law, privacy requirements, and other policies. |

# Appendix B. Key Publications and Programs

The materials listed here are suggested as sources for further information. Several of these documents were used to inform the development of the SPHM standards. This list is a highlight of available information and is not meant to represent a comprehensive list of available SPHM publications and programs. Many of these references are also cited throughout the document.

**American Nurses Association (ANA).** *The Elimination of Manual Patient Handling to Prevent Work-Related Musculoskeletal Disorders.* Within this position statement, ANA supports establishment of a safe environment of care for nurses and patients through actions and policies that result in the elimination of manual patient handling (ANA, 2008).

**American Nurses Association (ANA). Handle With Care® Program.** This educational campaign and online toolkit was developed by the ANA in response to nurses' concerns about injuries and MSDs (ANA, 2012a).

**Association of periOperative Registered Nurses (AORN).** *Safe Patient Handling Tool Kit.* AORN recognized the unique hazards faced by RNs in the surgical setting and developed a set of reference materials that can be helpful to any healthcare worker in the perioperative setting (AORN, 2012).

**Facilities Guidelines Institute (FGI).** *2010 Guidelines for the Design and Construction of Health Facilities.* FGI included both ergonomic design parameters and its Patient Handling and Movement Assessment (PHAMA) in these 2010 Guidelines (FGI, 2010a).

**Facilities Guidelines Institute (FGI).** *PHAMA White Paper.* The FGI published an white paper to accompany the *2010 Guidelines* to aid designers, engineers, and architects in understanding the need for and use of the PHAMA. The goal of this document was to guide project decision-makers toward the realization of SPHM throughout the nation's healthcare facilities (FGI, 2010b).

**House of Representatives (H.R.) 2381.** This bill was introduced into the 111th Congress as the Nurse and Healthcare Worker Protection Act of 2009 by Representative Conyers. The bill provides a strong framework for examining these issues. The purpose of the bill was to direct the Secretary of Labor to issue an occupational safety and health standard to reduce injuries to patients, direct-care registered nurses, and all other healthcare workers by establishing a safe patient handling and injury prevention standard (HR 2381, 2009). A companion bill was introduced into the Senate by Senator Franken. Both bills were referred to committee and died.

**International Organization for Standardization (ISO).** *Ergonomics: Manual Handling of People in the Healthcare Sector.* This document provides guidance to assess problems and risks associated with manual patient handling and mobility and identification and application of ergonomic strategies and solutions (ISO, 2012).

**The Joint Commission.** *Improving Patient and Worker Safety: Opportunities for Synergy, Collaboration and Innovation.* The purpose of this monograph is to increase awareness of the potential synergies between patient and worker health and safety. Included are a wide range of healthcare safety issues and tips for improving communication (JCAHO, 2012).

**National Institute for Occupational Safety and Health (NIOSH).** *Safe Patient Handling Nursing School Curriculum Module.* This resource, developed in partnership with the Veterans Health Administration (VHA) and ANA, provides evidence-based training to instructors at schools of nursing so that safe patient handling methods can be taught to students (NIOSH, 2009).

**National Institute for Occupational Safety and Health (NIOSH).** *Prevention through Design (PtD): Plan for the National Initiative.* The mission of the PtD National Initiative is to prevent or reduce occupational hazards by including prevention considerations in all designs that affect individuals in the occupational environment. This document outlines a national plan to implement PtD. Specific goals and activities in research, education, practice, policy, and business are included (NIOSH, 2010b).

**National Patient Safety Foundation.** *Through the Eyes of the Workforce: Creating Joy, Meaning, and Safer Health Care.* This report explores the current state of health care and outlines characteristics of a safe and healthy workplace. Seven recommendations of actions that organizations can take to effect real change are included in the document (NPSF, 2013).

**Occupational Safety and Health Administration (OSHA).** *Guidelines for Nursing Homes: Ergonomics for the Prevention of MSDs.* This resource outlines recommendations for nursing home employers. The recommendations are based on a review of existing practices and programs, state OSHA programs, and available scientific information (OSHA, 2009).

**U.S. Department of Veterans Affairs (VA).** *Safe Patient Handling and Movement Resource Page.* The VA Sunshine Healthcare Network maintains a web site with research and resources related to safe patient handling program implementation. Included are toolkits on bariatrics and slings, a technology resource guide, draft policies, and algorithms (VISN 8, 2013).

# References
# and Bibliography

Agency for Healthcare Research and Quality (AHRQ). (2012). *2011 national healthcare disparities and quality report.* Retrieved from www.ahrq.gov /qual/qrdr11.htm

Alamgir, H., Li, O., Gorman, E., Fast, C., Yu, S., & Kidd, C. (2009). Evaluation of ceiling lifts in health care settings: Patient outcomes and perceptions. *AAOHN Journal, 57*(9), 374–380.

American National Standards Institute (ANSI)/American Industrial Hygiene Association. (2005). American national *standard for occupational health and safety management systems.* New York: ANSI/AIHA. Retrieved from www.aiha.org/aihce07/handouts/po116palassis.pdf

American National Standards Institute (ANSI)/American Society of Safety Engineers (ASSE). (2011). *American national standard: Prevention through design—Guidelines for addressing occupational hazards and risks in design and redesign processes.* New York: ANSI/ASSE.

American Nurses Association (ANA). (2008). *The elimination of manual patient handling to prevent work-related musculoskeletal disorders.* Retrieved from http://nursingworld.org/MainMenuCategories /Policy-Advocacy/Positions-and-Resolutions/ANAPositionStatements /Position-Statements-Alphabetically/Elimination-of-Manual-Patient -Handling-to-Prevent-Work-Related-Musculoskeletal-Disorders.html

American Nurses Association (ANA). (2009, March 12). *Patient safety: Rights of registered nurses when considering a patient assignment.* Retrieved from http://nursingworld.org/rnrightsps

American Nurses Association (ANA). (2010). *Just culture.* Retrieved from http://nursingworld.org/psjustculture

American Nurses Association (ANA). (2011). *2011 health and safety survey.* Retrieved from http://www.nursingworld.org/MainMenuCategories /WorkplaceSafety/SafeNeedles/2011-HealthSafetySurvey.html

American Nurses Association (ANA). (2012a). *Handle with care.* American Nurses Association. Retrieved from http://www.anasafepatienthandling.org/

American Nurses Association (ANA). (2012b). *Principles for nurse staffing* (2nd ed.). Silver Spring: American Nurses Association.

Arnold, M., Radawiec, S., Campo, M., & Wright, L. (2011). Changes in functional independence measure ratings associated with safe patient handling. *Rehabilitation Nursing, 36*(4), 139–144.

Association of Occupational Health Professionals in Healthcare/OSHA. (2011). *Beyond getting started: A resource guide for implementing a safe patient handling program in the acute care setting.* Retrieved from http://www.aohp.org/About/documents/GSBeyond.pdf

Association of periOperative Registered Nurses (AORN). (2012). *Safe patient handling toolkit.* (A. o. Nurses, Producer). Retrieved from http://www.aorn.org/Secondary.aspx?id=20851&terms=safe%20patient%20handling#axzz2If9DxhGL

Association of Safe Patient Handling Professionals. (2012). *Learning center legislative updates.* Retrieved from http://www.asphp.org/learning-center/

ASTM International Committee E34.85. (2007). *Standard guide for integration of ergonomic/human factors into new occupational systems.* ASTM International. doi:10.1520/E2350-07

Australian Nurses Federation (Victorian Branch). (2009). *ANF nurses return to work in hospitals project, guidance on return to work duties.* Retrieved from http://www.nursesrtw.com.au/files/research/rtw_final_report.pdf

Brigham, C. (2010). Safe handling of residents in home health care. *Ergonomics in Design, 18*(1), 2628; doi:10.1518/1064804 10X12676454887224.

Bureau of Labor Statistics (BLS). (n.d.). *Occupational safety and health definitions.* Retrieved from http://www.bls.gov/iif/oshdef.htm

Bureau of Labor Statistics (BLS). (2011, November 9). *2010 nonfatal occupational injuries.* Retrieved from http://www.bls.gov/iif/oshwc/osh/case/osch0045.pdf

Bureau of Labor Statistics (BLS). (2012, November 8). *Nonfatal occupational injuries and illnesses requiring days away from work.* Retrieved from www.bls.gov/news.release/pdf/osh2.pdf

CAL/OSHA Consultation Service. (1997). *A back injury prevention guide for healthcare workers* (ed. M. Feletto & W. Graze). Retrieved from http://www.dir.ca.gov/dosh/dosh_publications/backinj.pdf

Centers for Disease Control and Prevention (CDC). (2010). *BRFSS maps 2010. Weight classification by body mass index.* Retrieved from http://apps.nccd.cdc.gov/gisbrfss/select_question.aspx

Centers for Disease Control and Prevention (CDC). (2011, January 27). *Healthcare associated infections (HAIs), laundry: Washing infected material.* Retrieved from http://www.cdc.gov/HAI/prevent/laundry.html and http://www.cdc.gov/hai/prevent/prevent_pubs.html

Centers for Medicare and Medicaid Services (CMS). (2013, March 21). *Pressure ulcers.* Retrieved from http://partnershipforpatients.cms.gov/p4p_resources/tsp-pressureulcers/toolpressureulcers.html

Charney, W. (2007). Nursing injury rates and negative patient outcomes: Connecting the dots. *AAOHN Journal, 55*(11), 470–475.

The Cincinnati Insurance Companies. (n.d.). *Return to work programs.* Retrieved from http://www.cinfin.com/Businesses_N_Organizations/Work_Comp/RTW_Programs.aspx

Cohen, M., Nelson, G., Green, D., Leib, R., Matz, M., & Thomas, P. E. (2010). *Patient handling and movement assessments: A white paper* (ed. C. Borden). Retrieved from www.fgiguidelines.org/pdfs/FGI_PHAMA_whitepaper_042810.pdf

Collins, J., Wolf, L., Bell, J., & Evanoff, B. (2004). An evaluation of a "best practices" musculoskeletal injury prevention program in nursing homes. *Injury Prevention, 10*(4), 206–211.

Collins, J. W. (2006). *Safe lifting and movement of nursing home residents.* Retrieved from www.cdc.gov/niosh/docs/2006-117/

CSP. (1962). *Lifting patients in hospital.* Retrieved from www.lancet.com/journals/lancet/article/PIIS0140

Darragh, A., Campo, M., Frost, L., Abernathy, N., Pentico, M., & Margulis, H. (2013). Safe patient handling technology in therapy practice: Implications for rehabilitation. *American Journal of Occupational Therapy 67*(1), 45–53.

Department of Health and Human Services (DHHS). (2010, July). *Access to medical care for individuals with mobility disabilities.* Retrieved from http://www.ada.gov/medcare_mobility_ta/medcare_ta.pdf

Enos, L. (2011). Making the business case to initiate, sustain, and evaluate safe patient handling programs: Part 1. *American Journal of Safe Patient Handling and Movement, 1*(3), 8–15. Retrieved from http://aasphm.org/resources /resource-library/making-a-business-case-for-sphm-programs/

Enos, L. (2011). Making the business case to initiate, sustain, and evaluate safe patient handling programs: Part 2. *American Journal of Safe Patient Handling and Movement, 1*(4), 8–16. Retrieved from http://www .americanjournalofsphm.com/shop_ajsphm/index.php?route=product /product&product_id=68

*Evidence-based behavioral practice.* (n.d.). Retrieved from www.ebbp.org

Facilities Guidelines Institute (FGI). (2010a). *Guidelines for design and construction of health care facilities.* Retrieved from http://www .fgiguidelines.org/

Facilities Guidelines Institute (FGI). (2010b). *Patient handling and mobility assessments: A white paper.* Retrieved from http://www.dli.mn.gov/WSC /PDF/FGI_PHAMAwhitepaper_042710.pdf

Food and Drug Administration (FDA). (2013, updated daily). *FDA: Safety, recalls, market withdraws and safety alerts.* Retrieved from http://www .fda.gov/safety/recalls/default.htm

Frankel, A., Leonard, M., & Denham, C. (2006). Fair and just culture, team behavior and leadership engagement: Tools to achieve high reliability. *Health Services Research, 41*(4, Pt. 2): doi:10.1111/j.1475-6773.2006.00572.x

Fryar, C., Carroll, M., & Ogden, C. (2012, September). *Prevalence of overweight, obesity, and extreme obesity among adults: United States, trends 1960–1962 through 2009–2010.* Retrieved from http://www.cdc. gov/nchs/data/hestat/obesity_adult_09_10/obesity_adult_09_10.pdf

Garg, A. (1999). *Long-term effectiveness of "zero-lift program" in seven nursing homes and one hospital*. Cincinnati, OH: NIOSH. Retrieved from http://www4.uwm.edu/ergonomics/research/upload/Zero-Lift_Report.pdf

Gucer, P. W., Gaitens, J., Oliver, M., & McDiarmid, M. A. (2013). Sit-stand powered mechanical lifts in long-term care and resident quality indicators. *Journal of Occupational and Environmental Medicine, 55* (1), 36–44.

Hampton, I. (1898). *Nursing: Its principles and practice*. Cleveland, OH: J. B. Savage.

Hannekom, S. E. (2011). *Clinical rehabilitation: The development of a clinical management algorithm for early physical activity and mobilization of critically ill patients*. SAGE. doi:10.1177/0269215510397677

Hignett, S. M., Fray, M. J., & Matz, M. (2012) Assessment and evaluation tools for health care ergonomics: Musculoskeletal disorders and patient handling. In P. Carayon (ed.), *Handbook of human factors and ergonomics in health care and patient safety* (pp. 235–246). Proceedings of the 2nd International Conference on Human Factors and Ergonomics in Healthcare/4th International Conference on Applied Human Factors and Ergonomics. CRC Press, Taylor and Francis Group.

HR 2381. (2009, May 13). *Nurse and health care worker protection act*. Retrieved from http://www.govtrack.us/congress/bills/111/hr2381/text

International Ergonomics Association. (2010). *What is ergonomics*. Retrieved from iea.cc: http://www.iea.cc/01_what/What%20is%20Ergonomics.html

Institute of Medicine (IOM). (2000). *To err is human: Building a safer health system*. Retrieved from http://www.nap.edu/openbook.php?isbn=0309068371

Institute of Medicine (IOM). (2008). *Retooling for an aging America: Building the health care workforce*.

Institute of Medicine (IOM). (2012). *Best care at lower cost: The path to a continuously learning healthcare system in America*. Retrieved from http://iom.edu/Reports/2012/Best-Care-at-Lower-Cost-The-Path-to-Continuously-Learning-Health-Care-in-America.aspx

International Organization for Standardization (ISO). (2004). *Ergonomic principles in the design of work systems.* Retrieved from www.iso.org/iso /catalogue_detail?csnumber=35885

International Organization for Standardization. (ISO). (2012). *Ergonomics: Manual handling of people in the healthcare sector.* Retrieved from www .iso.org/iso/home/store/catalogue.../catalogue_detail.htm

Jacobs, J. (2007). *Association law handbook* (4th ed.).Washington, DC: American Society of Association Executives.

Johns Hopkins Center for Innovation in Quality Patient Care. (n.d.). *Measuring culture of safety.* Retrieved from http://www.hopkinsmedicine .org/innovation_quality_Patient_care/areas_expertise/improve_Patient _safety/culture/measuring.html

The Joint Commission (TJC). (2001). *Healthcare at the crossroads: Strategies for addressing the evolving nursing crisis.* Retrieved from http://www.jointcommission.org/assets/1/18/health_care_at_the _crossroads.pdf

The Joint Commission (TJC). (2012). *Improving patient and worker safety: Opportunities for synergy, collaboration and innovation.* Oakbrook Terrace, IL: The Joint Commission. Retrieved from http://www .jointcommission.org

Montalvo, I. (2007). The National Database of Nursing Quality Indicators (NDNQI). *OJIN: The Online Journal of Issues in Nursing, 12*(3), Manuscript 2.

National Association for Home Care and Hospice. (n.d.). *NAHC store.* Retrieved from http://www.nahcstore.org /howtochooseahomecareagencyaconsumersguide.aspx

National Center for Health Statistics (NCHS). (2010). *National hospital discharge survey.* Retrieved from: http://www.cdc.gov/nchs/nhds.htm

National Fire Prevention Association (NFPA). (2000). *NFPA 101.* Author.

National Institute for Occupational Safety and Health (NIOSH). (2009). *NIOSH publications and products: Safe patient handling training for schools of nursing.* Retrieved from http://www.cdc.gov/niosh /docs/2009–127/

National Institute for Occupational Safety and Health (NIOSH). (2010a, January). *NIOSH hazard review: Occupational hazards in home health care* (DHHS NIOSH) Publication No. 2010-125). Retrieved from http: //www.cdc.gov/niosh/docs/2010-125/pdfs/2010-125.pdf

National Institute for Occupational Safety and Health (NIOSH). (2010b, November). *Prevention through design: Plan for the national initiative* (DHHS NIOSH) Publication Number 2011-121). Retrieved from http: //www.cdc.gov/niosh/docs/2011-121/pdfs/2011-121.pdf

National Institute for Occupational Safety and Health (NIOSH). (2010c). *Safe lifting and movement of nursing home residents.* Retrieved from http://www.cdc.gov/niosh/docs/2006-117/pdfs/2006-117.pdf

National Institute for Occupational Safety and Health. (2011, June 24). *Stop sticks campaign.* Retrieved from http://www.cdc.gov/niosh/stopsticks /safetyculture.html

National Institute for Occupational Safety and Health (NIOSH). (2012, December 18). *NIOSH program portfolio: Musculoskeletal disorders.* Retrieved from http://www.cdc.gov/niosh/programs/msd/

National Occupational Research Agenda (NORA). (2009, August). *State of the sector: Healthcare and social assistance—Identification of research opportunities for the next decade of NORA* (A NORA Report). Retrieved from http://www.cdc.gov/niosh/docs/2009-139/pdfs/2009-139.pdf

National Patient Safety Foundation (NPSF). (2013). *Through the eyes of the workforce: Creating joy, meaning, and safer health care.* Boston: Lucian Leape Institute at the NPSF.

National Quality Forum (NQF). (2013, March 21). *Effective communication and care.* Retrieved from http://www.qualityforum.org/Topics/Effective _Communication_and_Care_Coordination.aspx

Nelson, A. (2011). *Top 10 reasons why programs fail.* Paper presented at 11th Annual Safe Patient Handling & Movement Conference, Lake Buena Vista, FL. VISN 8 Patient Safety Center of Inquiry, U.S. Department of Veterans Affairs. Retrieved from http://www.visn8.va.gov /PatientSafetyCenter/safePtHandling/TopTen_Nelson.pdf

Nelson, A., & Baptiste, A. (2004). Evidence-based practices for safe patient handling and movement. *Online Journal of Issues in Nursing, 9*(3).

Nelson, A., Collins, J., Siddarthan, K., Matz, M., & Waters, T. (2008, January–February). Link between safe patient handling and patient outcomes in long term care. *Rehabilitation Nursing, 33*(1), 33–43.

Nelson, A., & Fragala, G. (2004). Technology for safe patient handling and movement. In W. Charney & A. Hudson (Eds.), *Back injury among healthcare workers* (pp. 121–135). Washington, DC: Lewis Publishers.

Nelson, A. F. (2003). Myths and facts about back injuries in nursing. *American Journal of Nursing, 103*(2), 32–40.

Nelson, A. L., Fragala, G., & Menzel, N. (2003). Myths and facts about back injuries in nursing. *American Journal of Nursing, 103,* 32–40.

Nelson, A. M., Collins, J., Chen, F., Siddharthan, K., Matz, M., & Fragala, G. (2008). Development and evaluation of a multifaceted ergonomics program to prevent injuries associated with patient handling tasks. *International Journal of Nursing Studies, 43*(6), 717–733.

Occupational Safety and Health Administration (OSHA). (2004). *OSHA forms for recording work related injuries and illness.* Retrieved from http://www.osha.gov/recordkeeping/new-osha300form1-1-04.pdf

Occupational Safety and Health Administration (OSHA). (2009, March). *Guidelines for nursing homes: Ergonomics for the prevention of musculoskeletal disorders.* Retrieved from http://www.osha.gov /ergonomics/guidelines/nursinghome/final_nh_guidelines.html

Occupational Safety and Health Administration (OSHA). (2013). *Healthcare facilities: Safe patient handling.* Retrieved from http://www.osha.gov/ SLTC/healthcarefacilities/safepatienthandling.html

O'Donnell, J. G.-S. (2011). An ergonomic protocol for patient transfer that can be successfully taught using simulation methods. *Clinical Simulation in Nursing,* e1–e12.

O'Donnell, J. G.-T. (2011). Effect of a simulation educational intervention on knowledge, attitude, and patient transfer skills: From the simulation laboratory to the clinical setting. *Simulation in Healthcare, 6*(2), 84–93.

Office of Human Resources Administration. (2006, January 24). *Department of Veterans Affairs workers' compensation strategic plan.* Retrieved from http:// www.va.gov/VASAFETY/WC_Strategic_Plan_Re_1_24_06.doc

Ontario Safety Association for Community and Healthcare. (2006). *Ergonomics in hospital design: A guide and workbook to prevent musculoskeletal disorders.* Retrieved from http://www .healthandsafetyontario.ca/PSHSA/Home.aspx

Pennsylvania Department of Labor and Industry. (n.d.). *Return to work: A model for Pennsylvania business and industry.* Retrieved from http:// www.portal.state.pa.us/portal/server.pt/community/return-to-work/1447

Pizzi, L., Goldfarb, N., & Nash, D. (2001). Promoting a culture of safety. In K. D. Shojana & K. E. McDonald (Eds.), *Making health care safer: A critical analysis of patient safety practices.* Rockville, MD: U.S. Agency for Healthcare Research and Quality. Retrieved from http://www.ncbi .nlm.nih.gov/books/NBK26959/ and http://www.ahrq.gov/clinic/ptsafety /chap40.htm

Radawiec, A. C. (2011, August). Changes in functional independence measure ratings associated with a safe patient handling and movement program. *Rehabilitation Nursing, 36*(4), 138–144. Retrieved from http://www.ncbi .nlm.nih.gov/pubmed/21721394

REBA. (2012). *Rapid entire body assessment.* Retrieved from http://www .ergo-plus.com/healthandsafetyblog/wp-content/uploads/2012/REBA-A -Step-By-Step-Guide.pdf.

Restrepo, T. S. (2013). Safe lifting programs at long-term care facilities and their impact on workers' compensation costs. *Journal of Occupational and Environmental Medicine, 55*(1), 27–35.

Salvendy, G. (2012). *Handbook of human factors and ergonomics* (4th ed.). Hoboken, NJ: John Wiley & Sons.

Snook, S. C., & Cierello, V. M. (1991). The design of manual handling tasks: Revised tables of maximum acceptable weights and forces. *Ergonomics, 34*(9), 1197–1213.

State Compensation Insurance Fund. (n.d.). *Return to work.* Retrieved from http://www.statefundca.com/claims/RTW.asp

Sturman-Floyd, M. (2012). "In-bed" systems can save money and cut injuries: Reducing the risk and incidence of pressure ulcers, manual handling loads, and carer-costs using "in-bed systems." *The Column: The Journal of the National Back Exchange, 24*(2), 16–22.

Texas 81st Legislature. (2009). *Goals: Legislative intent: General workers compensation: Mission of department* (The Resource Center, Work Comp Analysis Group). Retrieved from http://www .workcompanalysisgroup.com/end_content.php?id=3475&Doc_ ID=402.021&state=TX&sess_state=TX&regulation_cat=Texas%20 Statutes

Trinkoff, J. M. (2005). Staffing and worker injury in nursing homes. *American Journal of Public Health, 95*, 1220–1225.

Tullar, J. B. (2010). Occupational safety and health interventions to reduce musculoskeletal symptoms in the health care sector. *Journal of Occupational Rehabilitation, 20*(2), 199–219.

Veterans Health Administration (VHA). (2013). *Patient care ergonomic resource guide.* Retrieved from http://www.visn8.va.gov/VISN8 /PatientSafetyCenter/resguide/ErgoGuidePtOne.pdf

VISN 8 Patient Safety Center of Inquiry. (n.d.). *Algorithms for safe patient handling, mobility and movement.* Retrieved from http://www.visn8 .va.gov/visn8/patientsafetycenter/safePtHandling/default.asp

VISN 8 Patient Safety Center of Inquiry. (n.d.). *Bariatric toolkit.* Retrieved from http://www.index.va.gov/search/va/va_search.jsp?SQ=&TT=1&QT =Bariatric+toolkit&searchbtn=Search

VISN 8 Patient Safety Center of Inquiry. (n.d.). *Patient care slings selection and toolkit.* Retrieved from http://www.visn8.va.gov/visn8 /Patientsafetycenter/safePtHandling/default.asp

VISN 8 Patient Safety Center of Inquiry. (2005, Aug 31). *Patient care ergonomics resource guide: Safe patient handling.* Retrieved from http: //www.visn8.va.gov/patientsafetycenter/resguide/ErgoGuidePtOne.pdf

VISN 8 Patient Safety Center of Inquiry. (2013). *VA sunshine healthcare network.* Retrieved http://www.visn8.va.gov/patientsafetycenter /safepthandling/

Wardell, H. (2007). Reduction of injuries associated with patient handling. *AAOHN Journal, 55* (10), 407–412.

Warhola, C. (1980). *Planning for home health services: A resource handbook* (D. p. 80-14017). Washington, DC: U.S. Public Health Service.

Washington State Department of Labor. (n.d.). *Early return to work program*. Retrieved from http://www.lni.wa.gov/ClaimsIns/Insurance/Injury/LightDuty/Ertw/Default.asp

Waters, T. R. (2007). When is it safe to manually lift a patient? *American Journal of Nursing, 107*(8), 53–58.

Waters, T., Putz-Anderson, V., & Garg, A. (1994, January). *Applications manual for the revised NIOSH lifting equation*. Retrieved from http://www.cdc.gov/niosh/docs/94-110/pdfs/94-110.pdf

Wiener, M. J., & Tilly, J. (2002). Population ageing in the United States of America: Implications for public programmes. *International Journal of Epidemiology, 31* (4), 776–781.

World Health Organization (WHO). (2010). *Framework for action on interprofessional education and collaborative practice*. Geneva: World Health Organization. Retrieved from http://www.who.int/hrh/resources/framework_action/en/index.html

# Index

Frustration of healthcare workers, 22

Funding in SPHM programs, 17, 27

## G

"General Duty Clause," 18

*Guidelines for Nursing Homes: Ergonomics for the Prevention of MSDs*, 71

## H

Handle with Care Program, 8, 69

Handling and lifting
defined, 41
manual handling, elimination of, 7–8
safe lifting limits, 13–14

Hazards and hazardous conditions, 24, 50
reporting, 24, 47, 48, 50

Health Insurance Portability Privacy and Accountability Act, 38, 68

Healthcare organization
SPHM standards of care, 21–22
*See also* Organization

Healthcare population
U. S., demographics and characteristics, 8

Healthcare recipients
aging and, 8
defined, 41
obesity and, 2
U.S. population, 8
safety (*See* Safe patient handling and mobility (SPHM) programs)
*vs.* patient (terminology), 9

Healthcare systems, learning, 16

Healthcare workers
aging and, 8
comprehensive evaluation system, 38
culture of safety, 24
defined, 41
education, training, and maintaining competence, 31

frustration, 22
implementation of SPHM, 27
injuries, 1–2, 8
MSDs and, 1–2
obesity and, 2, 8
overexertion, 2
patient-centered SPHM assessment, 34, 35–36
SPHM standards of care, 21–22
SPHM technology, 30
*See also* Ancillary/support staff

High-risk tasks in SPHM, 27
defined, 41

Home care and home health issues, 14, 17, 25, 32
home care defined, 41–42
*See also* Plan of care

Home environments, 10
*See also* Environments of care; Home care

Hospital settings, 8, 9, 56

## I

Implementation of SPHM programs, 26–27
evaluative tools, strategies, resources, 49–52

*Improving Patient and Worker Safety: Opportunities for Synergy, Collaboration and Innovation*, 2, 70

Incidents (reporting), 24, 47, 48, 51, 67

In-patients, 9

Injuries, 1–2
age/obesity and, 2, 8
patient handling injury (defined), 42
post-injury return to work, 18, 43–44, 64–65
pushing/pulling motions and, 13
risk, physical fitness and, 14

Installation of SPHM technology
evaluative tools, strategies, resources, 55–57

# N

# O

# P